Primum non nocere

STORMS PASSING

What My Cancer Patients Taught Me About Living

MICHAEL L BERMAN, MD

WITH FOREWARD BY

KRISHNANSU S TEWARI, MD

BOHANNON HALL PRESS

Printed in the United States of America
First Edition

Cover Photo © by Michael L Berman

Library of Congress Control Number: 2024918526

Publisher's Cataloging-in-Publication Data
Berman, Michael L, 1942-
Storms Passing : What My Cancer Patients Taught Me About Living.
Foreward by Krishnansu S Tewari.
Niceville, Florida : Bohannon Hall Press, 2024
240 p. ; 23 cm.
First edition.
1. Oncologists—Personal Narratives. 2. Physicians' Writings—Nonfiction 3. Cancer-Women-Patients. 4. Physician and Patient.

"A career gynecologic oncologist shares his experiences for the benefit of aspiring young doctors and their patients."

RG104.6 B47 S76 2024 NLM WP660 B47 S76 2024 2024918526

ISBN 978-1-962995-04-7 (softcover)
ISBN 978-1-962995-07-8 (hardcover)

Published by Bohannon Hall Press

Composed for my grandchildren
Ben, Jack, Jake, Tyler, Ryan, Nathan, Anna and Samantha

And in memory of my wife, Marlene
Departed from our lives much too soon

Table of Contents

FOREWARD

A MEANINGFUL LIFE

Tyger Tyger, burning bright,
In the forests of the night;
What immortal hand or eye,
Could frame thy fearful symmetry?
William Blake

TORAH STUDY AND KABBALAH

When I consider Dr. Michael L. Berman's surgical philosophy, I must invoke *The Tyger* by England's great visionary and prophet, William Blake (1757-1827). A man whose life was spent on the fringes of Victorian Era London, Blake's writing and art petitions the mystical Jewish concepts of the Kabbalah. Dr. Berman always strove for perfection in the operating room to restore nature's *fearful symmetry* to organs and structures riddled with disease. In this respect, he channeled Kabbalistic methodology to gain a deeper understanding of what *was and was not* possible when treating women struggling with advanced gynecologic cancers.

I've known Dr. Berman for 29 years. The first ten years I was a 3rd and 4th year medical student, an Obstetrics & Gynecology Resident, and a Gynecologic Oncology Fellow. For the past 19 years he has been my professor, my mentor and a colleague. If someone had suggested back in the day that the future President of the Society of Gynecologic Oncologists (SGO) would later write what is essentially a moving tribute to his patients disguised as life lessons from a surgeon, I wouldn't have believed it. You see, "back in the day" was 1992 and I was a medical student. This was a time when Dr. Berman had been operating at the peak of his skills for over a decade and would continue to do so until his retirement in 2018. He was recognized for exceptional surgical technique and impossibly high surgical standards. He did not suffer fools gladly, and while he never lost his temper during surgery or on hospital rounds, I recall being terrified of him as a medical student.

Of course, the more time spent with a formidable giant, the more comfortable one becomes. Well, not quite. Dr. Berman strove for perfection in every facet of his professional life—from straight forward surgical procedures to highly complex, life-saving cancer operations. Patient interactions, scientific writing, lectures, review of clinical trials, health care expenditures and cost containment—all were fair game for the *Berman mental excavation* and dismantling into fundamental components to serve his overarching premise that excellence should always be pursued. If perfection proved elusive, it was not for lack of effort on his part. A former UC Irvine Fellow, Brad Monk, once said, "Mike Berman is the single most important critical thinker of our generation."

Armor and Sword

So, what exactly is this book and how does one distinguish it from his previous one from 2020? Well, on the surface, that's easy. The first, *Memories and Stories: 1942-2020* was a traditional autobiography laying out his life in more or less chronological fashion, providing a road map which connected the dots from childhood to Professor Emeritus and beyond. We've seen these books before, many are interesting, his was outstanding and a joy to read.

But *Storms Passing*, is not so easily described. On its surface, the stories contained herein are lessons that have shaped Dr. Berman's understanding of how life-threatening disease affects the patient, their families, and importantly, their doctor. There is that, but I believe, whether he is consciously aware of it or not, this book is also a long form love letter to his patients. The field of medicine, and especially, his immersion into the lives of his patients, has provided him with a full and meaningful life. Whereas the autobiography allows the reader an understanding of how he happened to get to wherever he was at different points of the narrative, this book places us in his mind's eye and allows us to understand why Dr. Berman could not be anyone other than who he is. I would imagine other successful surgeons could share a wealth of similar tales of patients whose journeys touched their lives, but to do this, those surgeons must have the capacity for self-appraisal and introspection and be willing to carve out the time to place fingers to keyboard.

Clearly, to write this book, there had to have been an interest in doing so; he must have been cast from some metallurgic alloy distinct from standard surgical stock. Some of this may be attributed to the importance (to him) of those beyond his immediate circle. While it's true that Dr. Philip J. DiSaia created the infrastructure of Gynecologic Oncology at UC Irvine, it was Dr. Berman who nurtured the concept of family.

Recall that I and others had been uncomfortable in his presence, fearing that we would fall short in his estimation, unable to perform to his high standards. But then I learned that he had gone to see the Rolling Stones in 1989 (in later years, when we compared notes, I realized it was one of the Coliseum shows in Los Angeles with Guns n' Roses as openers that I had also attended), and he was fond of bourbon (Gentleman Jack or Woodford Reserve, "neat" or with an ice cube to be accurate). Having great taste in live music and choice of evening beverage by no means distinguishes a surgeon, but at least it was something I could work with. I also came to know Dr. Berman outside the hospital environment when Fellows (Residents and Medical Students included) would be invited to his home for evening Journal Clubs with beer and pizza, bat mitzvahs (he has four daughters), annual Labor Day swim parties, and even the wedding of his daughter, Debbie, at Trentadue Winery in Sonoma County, and sadly when he would lay to rest his wife of 50 years, Marlene, in 2014. In return, he honored his trainees by attending weddings (mine, Julia Chapman, Noelle Cloven, Ellen Sheets in New Your City), and our parents' Celebrations of Life.

As a sidenote, I find it interesting how important first impressions are. Only recently, Dr. Berman had mentioned to my wife, Meagan, that "Krish is still afraid of me." Indeed, I remember in 2018 being at the top floor of the Bio Science Building to celebrate the creation of a scholarship in mine and my brother Devansu's parents' memory. Dr. Berman trained Devansu, also a gynecologic oncologist in Southern California. My back was to the elevator at the reception, and as its doors opened, I felt a chill along my spine and turned to see Dr. Berman and his girlfriend, Bonnie, stepping out to join the festivities. Devansu and I could sense his presence at the event before we knew that he had arrived.

Snakes and Ladders

In the pages that follow, Dr. Berman shares very personal stories of patients who are dear to him. It is not possible to come away from this book unmoved. Please indulge me, however, while I also share some anecdotes of what was taking place "behind the scenes." Since most of his operations were performed in hospitals assisted by Fellows and residents, there was a lot of teaching going on accompanied by his critical evaluation of our skills. Just as this book is rooted in morality lessons akin to Moksha Patamu—the primeval Indian board game that has come to be known as Snakes and

Ladders—the journey undertaken by Fellows at UC Irvine was punctuated by virtues (ladders) and vices (snakes), especially when operating with Dr. Berman.

There was not an operation for which each Fellow's surgical technique was not evaluated critically. Take the case of Katie, the patient from New Zealand. The assisting Fellow, Annie, recalled that during the operation she had made a potentially harmful move, but wasn't immediately called out for it. However, sure enough, seven or eight steps later, Dr. Berman chastised her for what had been done earlier, reminding her that "nothing is missed." Another Fellow, John Chan, was at the scrub sink getting ready to remove a bulky lymph node from the neck of Candy whose first encounter with cancer you'll be able to read about later. Dr. Berman leaned over to John and said, "we are about to embark on an area of the body that we don't visit often; accordingly, I am a little apprehensive." John thought to himself, thank God, he's human after all, when Dr. Berman leaned over a second time and said, "Not really."

Another time, a Fellow was operating with Dr. Berman on Joan whose story is also recalled quite vividly for her strength of character. Joan had relapsing disease and as the Fellow slowly chiseled away at the tumor, Dr. Berman's patience had reached its limit. "Ramez, when cancer has recurred, a patient is unlikely to be cured. But by removing this tumor we may be able to give her a few more years of life. However, if most of those years are spent in the operating room, we haven't really done her any favors."

There are different ways to teach—one is by nurturing as in the master-apprentice model, by which the professor recognizes the limitations of the students and carefully guides them, navigating the educational terrain. Sometimes handholding pays dividends. That was not his style. If you were assisting him in surgery, he believed that the patient deserved the best operation that could be performed and therefore he expected you to operate at his level of skill. All of his fellows and residents were reminded of this repeatedly over the years, none more so than me, but it was in an effort to improve our skills. I recall after seven years of working with him (four years of residency, three of fellowship) a particular incident. We operated on Janis, whose story is shared, with advanced ovarian cancer. Then we went to the infusion center to round on a couple of patients receiving chemotherapy and walked back to the OR for another case. He let me know during the walk that I was operating well, that I probably knew that, but he was sure that it was nice for me to hear it from him. I was thrilled and admitted it did feel good to hear him tell me that. Little would I know that would be the only complement on my surgical performance I would ever receive from him, even with an entire year left to train!

WHEEL OF DHARMA

Dr. Berman lets the reader know that former trainees will often ask of themselves during a difficult operation, "What would Dr. Berman do?" I can go one better—once I was in surgery assisting one of his former fellows, Bob Burger. We had gotten into some pretty heavy bleeding removing cancer from the inferior vena cava. As Bob prepared to suture this giant vessel, I could hear him mumbling. I couldn't make out the words and so I leaned over the table to listen carefully in case he was trying to give me instruction. This is what I heard, solemn as a prayer, a mantra: "Berman, be with me."

Indeed, with his first grandchild, Ben, fast asleep in the Presidential Suite of the Fontainebleau Hotel in Miami during the 2002 SGO Annual Meeting, Dr. Berman stepped to the podium to give his Presidential Address. The immediate Past President, Carolyn Runowicz, introduced him as having a reputation as the finest surgeon his trainees had ever worked with. This introduction was made before 1,000 attendees who were not laypersons or primary care physicians, but rather surgeons of the highest caliber and their oncology nurses. Strong praise indeed, which was likely to have resonated with the trainees in attendance, for it is common knowledge that no trainee is more hungry for surgery than Gynecologic Oncology Fellows...except, of course, if one considers Fabio Cappuccini's comments during Fellowship Graduation in 2002, "No one goes to the operating room with more passion every day than Dr. Berman."

By way of a brief interlude, I'd like to reference the cyclic nature of life. Remember that grandson, Ben, dreaming in Miami during his grandfather's Presidential Address? Now this kid is 20 years old, a pre medical student at Cornell, and is doing HPV and COVID-19 vaccine research under my mentorship. Derived from Sanskrit, the most ancient of languages. the Dharma Chakra continues to turn on the Buddhist Path of Enlightenment and Noble Eightfold Path...

Blood on the Tracks

Only a handful of stories are collected in this book, and hundreds more remain unchronicled. The intensity which fueled his patient encounters and provided the raw materials for his evolving societal and worldview, also *bled* into other integral components of academic life. For this reason, I need to segue briefly to his *tales of blood;* three of them, to be exact. First and foremost, we need to get it out of the way that Dr. Berman's surgical technique was so precise, so meticulous, so exacting, that there was hardly any blood loss in most of his cases. In fact, a common urban street legend held that Dr. Berman did not even know what color blood was! A permissible vascular injury, he said, had to be so tiny that red cells could escape from the injury in single file, scraping against the walls of the vessel. The second tale can stand up to testimony by any of his trainees. Whenever a scientific manuscript had been prepared and given over for his review and critique, it would be returned with so many red-lined corrections and substitutions that it would appear as if he had dipped a brush into a bucket of blood and splashed every word of every sentence on every page.

Tale #3 is one of personal recollection when I was practicing my oral ten-minute presentation for an upcoming Western Association of Gynecologic Oncologists Meeting. After 45 minutes of taking very difficult questions from Dr. Berman, I realized that I had not even gotten past slide #2. By then it was 6 pm and everyone had to leave; my presentation had literally been skewered and I was left bleeding at the podium. As Dr. Berman departed, he threw me a bone and suggested, "Better for this to have happened this afternoon among friends rather than in two weeks in front of a room full of Gynecologic Oncologists from around the country."

WONDROUS STORIES AND THE DARKNESS OF MERE BEING

In these pages Dr. Berman has immortalized his patients, many of whom are still going about their lives, cancer-free. Others contained herein have not been so fortunate. After reading this work, we discussed over e-mail the possibility of wider distribution beyond his intended audience (eight grandchildren). His reluctance is understandable as he was concerned that it would appear to be self-serving. On the contrary, I find it invigorating. Moreover, these wondrous stories demonstrate that it is still possible for the art of medicine to be practiced for the patient's sake alone. Amidst reduced reimbursement by Medicare, authorization constraints imposed by third party payors, and frivolous lawsuits, (all of which are discussed in the book), the patient and her sufferings sometimes take a back seat. I still remember spending two separate nights operating with Dr. Berman (on Christmas eve, and during Hanukkah) on undocumented unfunded women with non-oncologic conditions (necrotizing fasciitis, placenta accreta). We left the OR at 4 or 5 a.m. His only rewards were the patients' wellbeing. They were fine, and that was sufficient, as it should be.

As the progressive rock and new age songwriter Jon Anderson once sang, *If I was late, I had to leave to hear your wonderous stories.*

The book is also about faith but, interestingly, God is not discussed in these pages. I say interesting because the stakes are so high given that his patients have cancer—it is always a matter of life or death. He includes anecdotes concerning his patients' religious beliefs, as well as a deep appreciation for those who prayed for him, and respect for their religious beliefs, regardless of the faith they practiced.

Failing to reflect about God from the musings of a cancer surgeon may be understood in context. For example, "How can a merciful God permit innocent women to suffer so greatly?" There is no effort to address this unanswerable question. I suggest that one considers Monk's comment regarding Dr. Berman's critical insight in trying to understand his philosophical approach to this issue. Framed against the backdrop of more famous critical thinkers, a distinct theme emerges. Friedrich Nietzsche (1844-1900) is famously quoted for having stated that *God is dead,* but he was not "anti-religious;" rather, Nietzsche was a religious thinker who only rejected the Christian God. During their early friendship, Carl Jung (1875-1961) would quote Nietzsche in his letters to Sigmund Freud (1856-1939). Freud, himself a committed atheist of Hasidic Jewish background, readily acknowledged the important role religion would play in the development of the psychoanalytic school of thought. Meanwhile, in his later years, Jung's use of Kabbalistic symbols and ideas are nowhere more on display than in his assertion that "the sole purpose of human existence is to kindle a light in the darkness of mere being." To me, this summarizes Dr. Berman's own philosophy and what one finds on display here.

Songs of Innocence and of Experience

One story that is inconspicuous by its absence, of course, is the story of Marlene, his wife of 50 years. You can read all about her in the autobiography, but that book does not open doors into his psyche as do the other patient stories he writes about in this book. What was remarkable was that Dr. Berman operated on her when her breast cancer had recurred extensively in the pelvis. He resected bowel and a portion of her bladder, and she survived cancer-free for a decade afterwards, ultimately passing on, cancer free, due to complications from her autoimmune disease. I am reminded of Tom Hank's character, Captain John H. Miller, from the epic war film, *Saving Private Ryan.* During perhaps the one quiet moment in the movie before all Hell breaks loose, Ryan is sharing with Miller stories of his (now deceased) brothers. When Ryan asks Miller to tell him about his wife back at home and their rose garden, Miller declines to do so, saying that those memories are just for him.

Dr. Berman has remained in excellent health and has kept his mind sharp by playing sudoku, travelling the world, and maintaining a healthy and informed vantage point when it comes to American politics. As such, retirement has not allowed him to reinvent himself, but rather to move forward to the next exciting chapter that had always been pre-ordained. In addition to the aforementioned travels (which have included Antarctica, India, Japan, sub-Saharan Africa, and the Galapagos Islands), he has nurtured love and companionship with Bonnie, a passion for landscape and wildlife photography, and continues to discover new trails for wilderness hiking. Of course, he considers another great achievement to be his calculated escape from California's onerous state income tax laws by building a new home and moving to Incline Village, Nevada. And he has not remained idle on the medical forefront. He remains an active participant and discussant of the Gyn Oncology Division's monthly Academic Day sharing wisdom, medical-legal advice, and surgical philosophy when Fellows' surgical case logs are reviewed and scientific articles are presented. He hosts the quarterly Berman Book Club (these days by Zoom) for current and former Fellows, and, in the midst of the Pandemic, when resources were constrained and it was not clear whether health care providers would be dropping like flies, he called to volunteer his services for anything I felt would help.

And he also found the time to write his autobiography and this book. *Storms Passing* works on so many levels—for laypersons, for the patient, for their families, but also for trainees, perhaps especially trainees excited by the prospects of going out and having their own patients to care for and impact their lives. The book also resonates with practicing physicians, many of us who might have become slightly cynical or even jaded. I can honestly say reading this book rejuvenated me and I am able, once again, to appreciate many things about the practice of medicine and oncology that I may have forgotten, unlike Dr. Berman, who never lost his way and has always remained true to his guiding principles. There's a lot going on here.

I will close by citing a portion of William Blake's patriotic poem, *Jerusalem,* published in 1804 and adopted as a kind of alternative national anthem for England. In this poem from which, incidentally, the title of the movie *Chariots of Fire* was named, Blake invokes a call to arms with the famous words: *I will not cease from Mental Fight, Nor shall my sword sleep in my hand.* These words epitomize Dr. Berman's vision of rising to the challenge of fighting life's battles for his patients as chronicled in *Storms Passing.* It is a worthy ending of my Foreward and tribute to this most enjoyable and readable text.

Krishnansu S. Tewari, MD, FACOG, FACS, FRSM

Professor and Division Director
The Philip J. DiSaia Chair in Gynecologic Oncology
Division of Gynecologic Oncology
Department of Obstetrics & Gynecology
University of California, Irvine

CHAPTER ONE

THE BEGINNING

I wrote a book once. It was an autobiography. I read it after I wrote it, and I thought it was pretty good. I hope my children and grand-children will read it someday to know a little bit about me they didn't know previously. They might even think my life was interesting and memorable. Maybe not, but I hope so. Then I thought, I have a lot of free time, so what could I write as an encore that would give all of them more insight into their dad and grandpa? Could I teach them some of life's lessons I've learned over my many years? What could I write?

Well, I *am* a doctor, and doctors have a wealth of opportunities to impact the lives of others. And then, I am also a gynecologist. And as a gynecologist, I had been instrumental in the lives of lots of women and their families. But I am also a cancer doctor for women, so I had an effect on women and their families at times in their lives when they were facing their own mortality. Was there an opportunity to make observations that would be important to my family and help explain why I did what I did? Why I chose this career path? Could I create a sense of how much I have loved what I've done professionally for 42 years as a practicing gynecologic oncologist? I hope so. That is the purpose of this, my second book.

First, I wanted to explain how I went from being a medical student at George Washington University School of Medicine as an incoming freshman on September 3, 1963, to becoming a gynecologic oncologist on June 30, 1976. That was nearly 13 years of my life during a time when many of my friends from high school and college were working and earning a nice living. They were taking fancy vacations in exotic distant locations, buying nice houses, and living the good life. For 13 years I was a student, four years in medical school, one year of internship in Denver, Colorado, a year of residency in obstetrics and gynecology, all followed by two years in the Commissioned Corps of the U.S. Public Health Service.

Then there were three more years of obstetrics and gynecology residency at Harbor UCLA Medical Center and then two years as a fellow in gynecologic oncology at UCLA and the City of Hope.

This was years before gynecologic oncology fellowships required a three- or four-year commitment with at least one year in the laboratory as a cancer researcher. I'm not certain I would have been interested in a fellowship that was longer than two years; however, that was not a requirement in the mid 1970's.

When I became a medical student, I had no idea which field of medicine I wanted to pursue. I knew I wanted to take care of sick patients and thought a surgical field would be exciting, but I really had no idea where my career would go.

My only role model growing up was my family physician, Dr. Jacob Ceppos, who had a solo family practice in Washington, DC. "Dr. Jack" worked out of his home office. He was quiet and rarely smiled, but he seemed to know just about everything about sick patients and how to keep healthy people from getting sick. He did physical examinations, administered inoculations to prevent diseases and made referrals when necessary. He even made house calls, especially when I was sick with acute glomerulonephritis as a ten-year-old in the 6th grade. I don't think I admired him particularly then or thought I wanted to be like him. He was just Dr. Jack, our family doctor.

I'd like to say that was my entire exposure to medicine when I was growing up except that I also had a ventral hernia repair at Providence Hospital in Washington, DC when I was about eight or nine years old. Looking back, I am pretty sure it was a lipoma rather than a ventral hernia. I recall being asymptomatic and, later in life I developed familial multiple lipomatosis (FML) which I inherited from my father. Today, I probably have more than a hundred lipomas on my trunk and extremities. I think this was just an early manifestation of that condition.

I don't know for sure that I would have gone into medicine if my mother, the prototypical Jewish matriarch, had not encouraged me to do so from the time I was a young boy. I was not a strong student in English and had not demonstrated any aptitude for the sciences prior to my senior year in high school. I knew that doctors were really smart and so, of course, I assumed that they must have gotten excellent grades in school. When I was in high school, with just above average but not outstanding grades, I figured I probably could not be a doctor. To my way of thinking, my grades didn't seem to be good enough to compete with students who wanted to be doctors. And there were certainly other students who seemed to be a lot smarter than I was. The areas where I really stood out were in mathematics at every level of high school (algebra I and II, geometry, trigonometry and calculus) and chemistry as a senior in high school. I loved inorganic chemistry largely because it involved a lot of mathematics and chemical equations. I was the strongest student in my chemistry class.

When my friends in high school asked me what I was going to do when I became an adult, I told them I would be "a dentist" because it was a medical field and I figured you didn't need such high grades to get into dental school. I was pretty naïve about that. It is just as hard to get into dental school as it is into medical school these days, and probably was back then as well. So anyway, somewhere along the way, I decided to "go for it" and see if I could get into medical school even though I didn't think I was the brightest or most intellectual of my peers.

I had a lot of friends in high school who tended to be less than academic superstars, so they thought I was "a brain" but I didn't necessarily agree with them. My good friend, Norman Brickman, was an exception among my friends and seemed to be much smarter than I was. I didn't have this special calling to medicine, I just liked the idea of helping people and I knew that doctors lived comfortably. The idea of helping people and living comfortably seemed like worthy goals. So, I worked hard at the University of Maryland and achieved passably good grades as a physical sciences major with an emphasis on mathematics and chemistry. I was accepted to all three medical schools I applied to (George Washington, Georgetown, and University of Maryland) with a grade point average just above 3.0. Today, I wouldn't even be considered for an interview, with such a meager grade point average, but A's were a lot harder to get 60 years ago than now. I wrote extensively about grade inflation that exists today in school at all levels of education in my autobiography. Teachers really didn't care if they hurt your feelings by giving you a poor grade in those days and you could never convince a teacher to give you a better grade than you deserved. Basically, you received the grade you earned based upon performance on the tests given. My grandchildren cannot fathom how I got grades that are pretty average by today's standards since, just like my peers in high school, they seem to think I am really smart. In any case, I enrolled into The George Washington University School of Medicine just after Labor Day, in September 1963.

The first two years at George Washington were the "basic sciences." These courses included anatomy, biochemistry, physiology, pharmacology, microbiology, and pathology, but there was no interaction with patients or the doctors who took care of patients. The professors were PhD's in their respective fields and not MD's. Lack of early patient contact was the standard for early medical education, and I was not surprised. Modern medical education today often incorporates patient contact much earlier than was typical when I was in school. Intuitively I understood that the basic sciences would provide the foundation for patient care which would follow. These courses would help me understand the hows and whys of human diseases. I understood that it would all fit together somehow, someday, much as organic chemistry prepares a future researcher for a life working on vaccines for viral illnesses or how basic physics links to electrical engineering.

Late in my second year of medical school I was assigned an obstetrical patient to follow during her pregnancy along with her private obstetrician. She was going to deliver at The Washington Hospital Center in Washington, DC. I met her in her second trimester of pregnancy, was an observer of her progress during her third trimester and was notified by her obstetrician when she went into labor. I had never attended a labor or a delivery. I didn't know exactly what to expect, but I was very interested in the process and very excited for this mom to be.

This was the first real patient in whose care I participated, although I do recall measuring fellow students' blood pressure, listening to their hearts and lungs and palpating their abdomens in the second year.

The labor and delivery were uneventful, and I was even allowed to assist in the delivery of the infant and cut the umbilical cord. For me it was an enchanting experience then, and even now as I think back to that delivery nearly 60 years ago. Everyone was excited and happy including the mom, the dad, the obstetrician and, of course, me. Up to that point in my life it was one of the most memorable events I had experienced. I didn't decide then and there that I wanted to become an obstetrician, but I certainly didn't rule out that possibility going forward.

The third year of medical school was what I had eagerly anticipated from the moment I was first accepted. I was participating in patient care as a member of the medical team. I didn't mind doing all the scut work medical students had to do in those days such as drawing blood, starting IVs, calling for laboratory results, running to the radiology department for X-rays, etc. Nowadays these tasks are typically done by medical assistants, nurses, and the phlebotomy team rather than medical students. The sophisticated computer software employed today provides laboratory results and X-ray results online within minutes of their being completed. Medical students these days are treated much kindlier than when I was in medical school. Some observers have said that students are babied, but I think the changes have been humane and in the spirit of improving medical education. Students no longer must run around as if their hair is on fire to find the results of the many tests ordered on their patients.

I should mention that many of those tests ordered then and now are often unnecessary, repetitive or redundant, but there often is little oversight of laboratory studies, X-rays and even some procedures ordered by trainees. Furthermore, in most settings, there is little motivation of supervising faculty to control the wasteful use of resources in providing care to our patients. As a result, CT scans are often ordered when an inexpensive plain film of the abdomen will provide the required information, repetitive X-rays are ordered sometimes daily when careful auscultation of the chest or examination of the abdomen would be sufficient, and the list goes on. Good clinical judgement based upon a careful history and physical exam often is replaced by a battery of tests that are often costly and unnecessary.

There were many highs and a few lows during my training to become a physician; however, I was happy with my decision to become a doctor, especially once I was in my third year of medical school. It was truly fascinating. Exposure to surgery, internal medicine, obstetrics and gynecology, psychiatry, pediatrics, family practice and the various medical and surgical specialties provided a series of adventures for me. The spectrum of diseases that I saw in the inpatient and the outpatient setting, and the variety of treatments that were employed by the treating physicians were mind-opening to this medical neophyte. I just had to decide what field of medicine I wanted to join. As with most medical students, this important decision was not an easy one.

It was easy for me to eliminate psychiatry because I was skeptical that psychiatrists really helped many of their patients. I was even told by someone (likely not a psychiatrist) that of patients who see a psychiatrist, a third get better, a third stay about the same and a third get worse. I didn't like those odds. Furthermore, somehow, I could not wrap my arms around the concept that most emotional problems were real diseases. Sure, I understood that schizophrenia and bipolar disease were "real diseases." However, I knew that most patients seen by psychiatrists had a myriad of complaints that were not easily compartmentalized or identified as "diseases." I have certainly come a long way since then, and I admire greatly the help that psychiatrists (and now, generations later, psychologists and social workers) provide their patients. In fact, in my professional career, I think one of the most valuable aspects of the care I provide is the listening and counseling of the patients and family members I treat. I believe that it is not possible to be an effective and caring physician without the ability to embrace listening skills and counseling techniques I learned about on my psychiatric rotation in medical school.

The second reason I excluded psychiatry as a career choice is that I liked the idea of using my hands in my practice of medicine. Surgical procedures, obstetrical deliveries, etc. seemed like a better fit for me. In any case, psychiatry was the easiest of the medical fields for me to eliminate as I looked to choose a medical career for myself. My exposure to psychiatry was a six-week rotation at St Elizabeth's Hospital in Washington, DC where a lot of very sick institutionalized patients were cared for. I didn't have much direct exposure to the patients there and most of my learning was in the classroom. Perhaps if I had direct exposure to those patients, my opinions might have been different; however, I doubt it.

Second to psychiatry, I easily eliminated pediatrics from consideration. I understood the concept that children are not just little people and that their diseases and treatments are very different from those seen in adults. Still, I thought pediatric care for babies and toddlers was a lot like veterinarian medicine where the patient could be quite sick but generally not able to communicate with the physician using normal language skills. I believed what my professors had taught me, that the most important tool to evaluate a patient with a medical problem is taking a careful history. That does not work so well with a wailing infant and a distraught mom. Furthermore, I knew that most of pediatrics was pretty humdrum largely consisting of wellness exams, vaccinations, rashes, acne, runny noses, sprains and cuts, and a host of really boring stuff. The interesting part of pediatrics, such as childhood cancers, were awful to deal with, because in those days you could not cure many of them. In addition, the interesting cases were the ones you had to refer to someone else to evaluate and manage.

I should note, however, that the poor prognosis for childhood cancers has changed dramatically since I was a medical student, with high cure rates for the most common of them. Just reading a fabulous book, *The Emperor of All Maladies* by Siddhartha Mukherjee, gives one a sense how far medicine has come in understanding and effectively treating many cancers, especially those seen in childhood. Furthermore, in reciting my decision to exclude pediatrics from my professional future is the understanding that it is a specialty without much opportunity to do procedures, unless one becomes a pediatric surgeon. Frankly, I was not really interested in caring for infants, toddlers, young children, and adolescents. I love them as my own children and continue to enjoy seeing my grandchildren become young adults; however, I didn't want to take care of them as their physician. My six-week rotation at the Children's National Hospital in downtown Washington, DC was less than exciting for me and confirmed my preconceived notion that I did not want to be a pediatrician.

I also excluded family practice and internal medicine for the same reasons I mentioned above; I wanted to do things with my hands. That left only the surgical specialties. I had excluded radiology, for example, because at that time the radiologists had limited patient contact. And the specialty of interventional radiology, in which today, the radiologist performs amazingly intricate lifesaving procedures, was not even envisioned.

This specialty has become one of the most important ones in the management of serious medical illnesses. The interventional radiologist can often eliminate the need for surgical procedures to stop uncontrollable bleeding almost anywhere in the body, save a damaged organ like the kidney or liver and even manage potentially lethal conditions affecting the blood vessels in the heart and brain. It is a truly remarkable specialty that has evolved only over the past twenty-five years. In fact, the American Board of Radiology first recognized Interventional Radiology as a unique medical specialty only in 2012 although the practice of the specialty preceded that date by more than a decade. When my wife, Marlene, suffered extraordinarily painful fractures in her spine, an interventional radiologist (interventional neuroradiologist to be precise) was able to stabilize the fractures and relieve her pain without surgical intervention. It was simply amazing that the minimally invasive procedure allowed her to avoid a potentially dangerous back operation with a long recovery and an uncertain outcome.

Similarly, I excluded pathology as a field for my pursuit because of the lack of patient contact, even though I loved pathology and do so to this day. Pathologists are the super sleuths who can uncover a myriad of mysteries by evaluating human tissues. Is a tumor benign or cancerous? Do the features of this cancer suggest a good prognosis or a poor one? Based on a biopsy alone, can I discern whether this woman ovulated or not last month? Are the cells on this Pap smear worrisome or reassuring? What type of infection is this, anyway? So many questions asked by clinicians are answered by the pathologist.

I easily excluded the myriad of medical specialties of dermatology, gastroenterology (nowadays these physicians spend all their time doing procedures, colonoscopy, upper endoscopy, etc.), nephrology, neurology, and so on, which were basically non-surgical endeavors. The bottom line is that I wanted to be a surgeon, but one who also was knowledgeable about various nonsurgical medical specialties. To my way of thinking, many of the best physicians were surgeons of one type or the other. I loved stories of great surgeons such as Halstead, Cushing, Kelly, and others, who developed breakthrough operations to save lives or improve the quality of life for their patients. I believed the assertion that a great surgeon is like a trained internist who also has the skills to operate. I loved the idea that I could be knowledgeable about the field of internal medicine and also be able to help my patients and cure diseases surgically. So, in short, that left Obstetrics and Gynecology and many other surgical specialties for me to consider when making a choice of a medical field for my career.

CHAPTER TWO

CHOOSING A SPECIALTY

So, how did I choose Obstetrics and Gynecology over general surgery, or cardiothoracic surgery, or orthopedics, or neurosurgery, or plastic surgery, or the myriad of other surgical specialties? It turns out it was a rather easy decision for me. Physicians often choose a specialty wherein their experience as a medical student was especially positive and enjoyable. My clinical rotation on obstetrics at the District of Columbia General Hospital was exciting. I got to manage a lot of women in labor and was fortunate to deliver several infants. I even applied forceps to a couple of women to facilitate their deliveries under the watchful eyes of my resident. I managed magnesium sulfate infusions for women with severe preeclampsia. I helped pregnant diabetics control their blood sugars. I learned about the physiological changes that are unique to pregnancy. And I felt like a real doctor. The service was run by senior residents. There was little faculty involvement for these indigent women. Still, their management was delivered with care and was pretty much free of complications.

I had no exposure to most of the surgical specialties and therefore I just could not relate to them. No plastic surgery, ophthalmology, neurosurgery (although I knew that neurosurgical procedures could last 12-15 hours, sometimes as emergencies in the middle of the night, so that was an easy one to exclude), or orthopedics for that matter. I did see a lot of general surgery at the George Washington University Hospital. I recall there were some real characters in the general surgery department.

There was Dr. Brian Blades, with a name that screamed "you were born to be a surgeon." He was a surgeon's surgeon and widely recognized for his academic and surgical achievements. Dr. Blades was professor and chairman of the Department of Surgery and had been the 37th president of The American Association for Thoracic Surgery. He had even assisted at surgery on President Dwight D. Eisenhower in 1956 at Walter Reed Army Medical Center. He was a chain-smoking cardiothoracic surgeon who removed the diseased lungs of patients with cancer caused by smoking cigarettes. He died from a stroke many years later in 1977 undoubtedly related to his own nicotine addiction.

And there was Dr. Alec Horowitz, a diminutive 60-year-old Napoleonic type who preferred barking at you rather than speaking to you. But he was an amazing general surgeon. I remember holding retractors for him during an operation and he kept saying "pull harder." I kept pulling harder until finally he said, "easy boy" because I was pulling so hard that I was moving the patient on the OR table. I was able to assist him on several operations that were straightforward, but, at the time, I thought they were amazing.

I loved general surgery and gave it some consideration; however, I chose Obstetrics and Gynecology anyway. I had performed well in Obstetrics as a student. (I was elected president of the Obstetrical honor society "Kane King Society." More on that later.) I loved the secrets that gynecologic pathology uncovered. I loved the joy obstetrics brings to its patients most of the time, although sometimes it can be incredibly sad and depressing. And I viewed the field of Obstetrics and Gynecology as narrow enough that I believed that I could master the field. I could see myself possibly becoming a star within the specialty.

Frankly, the field has become so specialized over the past half century that no one can master the entire spectrum of obstetrics and gynecology, but in those days a diligent physician could. It was basically obstetrics and general gynecology without any specialized training available beyond a 3- or 4-year residency. The doctors of obstetrics and gynecology (OB/GYN) did the cancer operations, although poorly. They managed infertility with little success. And they managed urinary complaints surgically with no real understanding of the pathophysiological basis for their patients' complaints. Women with stress incontinence typically underwent a vaginal hysterectomy with a "bladder repair" that rarely was very helpful and often worsened the patients' symptoms. Ultrasound and fetal monitoring were on the horizon; however, not available when I was a medical student. Interestingly, fetal monitoring was being used widely in obstetrics by the time I was in my residency and has had a dramatic positive effect on neonatal outcome. There were lots of vaginal births, some C-sections, many hysterectomies, and other procedures. This was the typical practice of an OB/GYN when I was a resident.

I remember the first cancer operation I observed being done by the chairman of the department of obstetrics and gynecology at George Washington University Hospital in 1969 while I was a first-year resident. It was a radical vulvectomy for vulvar cancer. The procedure took about five hours to complete. There were several units of blood loss (a unit of blood is approximately a pint) and in hindsight, the operation was a total mess. I didn't know much about oncological surgery then, but I sure knew that there had to be a better way to manage this woman's cancer. (Typically, now the operation for vulvar cancer takes about 90 minutes and blood loss is usually minimal.) Looking back over these memories, I guess it's not so obvious why

I was motivated to become an OB/GYN; however, it seemed like a natural choice for me at the time.

Nowadays there are numerous subspecialties of Obstetrics and Gynecology that did not exist when I was a medical student. These fields include Maternal Fetal Medicine, Complex Family Planning, Reproductive Endocrinology and Infertility, Female Pelvic Medicine and Reconstructive Surgery, Pediatric and Adolescent Gynecology and, of course, Gynecologic Oncology. None of these existed back in the 1960s when I was in school, so, I believed that mastery of the specialty of Obstetrics and Gynecology was within my reach. Furthermore, I had the sense that improvements in the care of these women were on the horizon and I hoped to be a part of that change.

I should state now that if I had my career to do over, it might have been a more difficult choice. I always wanted to do well financially, but more important to me than doing well was to do good. If I were a medical student today, I would consider Interventional Radiology and Plastic Surgery in addition to Gynecologic Oncology. I already explained why Interventional Radiology is such an exciting field. My attraction to it should be evident from my description above. I also love plastic surgery and can envision myself having done a general surgery residency followed by training in plastic surgery.

When one thinks of plastic surgery, typically one envisions the lucrative cosmetic surgery that rewards the physician so handsomely. Plastic surgeons live in the mansions on the top of the hills overlooking the ocean, or near beautiful lakes or mountains. Much of their wealth results from cosmetic procedures they perform, always paid for in advance, typically by well-heeled patients who never die of their disease, because there is usually no disease being treated. Unlike physicians in most medical fields, plastic surgeons do not have to fight with insurance companies just to get paid a small percentage of their usual fees. That observation alone helps explain my attraction to the field. But as a reminder of doing *well* versus doing *good*, the real attraction of plastic surgery for me is reconstruction that restores functioning limbs, replaces missing body parts, covers genetic defects or traumatic wounds. Reconstructive plastic surgical procedures include facial reconstruction, burn management, microvascular procedures, and so on. In plastic surgery, the physicians can make such a difference in the lives of their patients by performing reconstructive cutting-edge surgery, while also being rewarded financially with their cosmetic work. Of course, when I was in medical school, plastic surgeons mostly did cosmetic surgery. The exciting reconstructive surgery was in its infancy having evolved from the surgical management of wounds sustained on the battlefield largely during the second world war.

I do not mean to suggest that plastic surgeons are the only ones who live in mansions on mountains or overlooking the ocean. I should mention their neighbors: orthopedists, ophthalmologists (the ones who do lots of laser procedures and cataracts) and, surprisingly often, dermatologists to name just a few of the more lucrative fields of medicine. Oh, by the way, radiation therapists and medical oncologists, who often participate in the care of cancer patients, also do very well financially.

Let me stop and take a moment to apologize for my comments about compensation of highly remunerated physicians. I am afraid I'll leave a sense of negativity about physicians who choose those fields. I would be remiss if I didn't point out that there are far easier ways to become wealthy than by becoming a physician: starting your own business, becoming an attorney (especially in plaintiff malpractice), or entering into wealth management. Inheritance works, too, but that is another story. Frankly, becoming a physician is hard work, as I will emphasize throughout this book. It deserves fair compensation although health insurance payers often seem to disagree with this premise. Most importantly, as I hope you will agree, all that hard work is well worth the effort.

But I digress. I chose a residency in Obstetrics and Gynecology for all the reasons I outlined above. I thought being an OB/GYN physician would be fulfilling and rewarding; however, there were pieces of the puzzle I had not considered. First, Obstetrics is great fun unless you must awaken from a peaceful sleep between 12:30 and 4:30 a.m. for an uncomplicated delivery. Then, it is not so enjoyable, especially for someone like me who has always had a difficult time falling back to sleep after being awakened. Furthermore, office gynecology, which is a mainstay of most practices, consists largely of well woman exams, birth control administration, vaginal discharge, hormone replacement therapy, and a whole lot of complaining women with family issues related to work, adolescent kids, wayward husbands, etc. They all find the need to share everything with their gynecologist. That's a big part of the typical practice in the specialty of Obstetrics and Gynecology.

Furthermore, while Obstetrics is joyful 99.5% of the time it is an absolute nightmare 0.5% of the time when a baby dies or is injured during labor or delivery, a baby with a serious malformation is delivered or the mom has some awful complication. Then the second guessing begins, and one doubts oneself for decisions made. That is also when plaintiffs' attorneys tell you what a piece of shit you are and when malpractice consulting doctors opine on what you should have done differently to achieve a better outcome.

I should note that discussing such sensitive issues as poor bladder control, menopausal symptoms, vaginal discharge, birth control needs, etc. with a physician is incredibly difficult for many women, and even more so when that physician is a male. This helps to explain why women now make up the large majority of OB/GYN physicians today. I believe that female physicians often are more sensitive to the psychosocial needs and concerns of their patients than their male counterparts, and that female physicians often relate better to their female patients than male physicians. Certainly, this is not a paradigm. Just as there are many male physicians who effectively meet all the psychosocial needs of their female patients, there are many female physicians who do not. Still the shift from a male dominated specialty which existed when I did my residency to one where nearly 90% of OB/GYN residents today are female is easily understood.

In this book, I elected to exclude my experiences as a first-year resident at George Washington University (other than my observation of a radical vulvectomy mentioned above), my two years of military obligation in the Public Health service at the National Institutes of Health and in Alaska, and my final three years of residency at Harbor UCLA Hospital in Torrance, California. I recounted all these experiences in my autobiography entitled "Memories and Stories - 1942 to 2020." So, let me continue my story with my 4th year of residency as a Chief Resident at Harbor UCLA Hospital.

When I was a senior resident, two important events occurred. First, I was chief resident on the Obstetrics service for three months. This time will forever be known as a *reign of terror* in the hallowed halls of Harbor UCLA Hospital. There were more complications during those three months than over the rest of the year through no fault of my own. Residents have a great deal of autonomy in the management of their patients; however, there is a high level of supervision by the faculty to prevent residents from making serious errors. I had appropriate supervision and just an incredible amount of bad luck. There were infants requiring care in the neonatal ICU, hemorrhaging mothers, and severe obstetrical infections. The list goes on. Even before my chief residency experience on the obstetrical service, I knew I didn't want to practice routine obstetrics or office gynecology when I finished my training. If I ever had a doubt, this three-month rotation convinced me. I needed to find a niche that worked for me.

That brings me to the second career-directing event which was my rotation at the City of Hope National Cancer Center in Duarte, California. I really loved it and thrived there. I operated with general surgeons on the staff of the City of Hope as well as the gynecologic oncologists from UCLA who provided care for women with pelvic malignancies. I got to assist and perform major portions of operations that included removing the stomach, or the colon, a kidney or a breast or a thyroid gland with the staff general surgeons. I also helped perform all the operations one can imagine on women with gynecologic cancers with the gynecologic oncologists from UCLA. The oncologic surgeons there were so good they made me look as if I was doing the operations myself. Of course, they were in complete control. The UCLA faculty who ran the gynecologic oncology program loved me and wanted me to become their gynecologic oncology fellow beginning in July 1974. I wrote all about this in my autobiography; however, the bottom line is I accepted their offer.

I spent the next two years, initially at the City of Hope as a first-year fellow and then at UCLA Medical Center as a second-year fellow in gynecologic oncology. Over those two years I learned to function independently as a gynecologic oncologist. I was given progressively increasing responsibility to make life and death decisions as a member of the gynecologic oncology team, and to perform complex cancer operations with oversight by faculty. On June 30, 1976, I matriculated as a gynecologic oncologist and began my career as a faculty member in the division of gynecologic oncology at UCLA. I was an assistant professor under the direction of Leo D. Lagasse, MD, my mentor, a true gentleman, one of the kindest men I have ever known, and a pioneer in the development of the specialty.

CHAPTER THREE

THE PATIENTS

Gynecologic Oncology is an amazingly fulfilling specialty for any physician embarking on a career in medicine. Ask most gynecologic oncologists. They will tell you it's because of the patients. The patients are the best. Their strength of character, their ability to deal with serious disease and even impending death with dignity is remarkable. They set a standard for courage and heroism that is difficult to match. I have written this book in large part to honor these heroic women. I would like to honor them by sharing my memories of a few of them whom I have cared for over the years. There have actually been at least ten thousand on whom I have operated. There were many more I provided care for who did not require surgery. Given the large number of patients I have seen and provided care, I know in advance that my recall of many details of the cases I will share will be imperfect. Still, I want to pass on some of the stories of the many women who have honored me by entrusting me with their lives. What an honor, what a responsibility.

Every life is important and has value. Everyone has loved ones who care for them and care about them. For the survivors, every life lost to cancer or any devastating disease causes pain for years to come. Premature loss of life means not seeing a child reach adulthood, getting married and having children. It means not seeing grandchildren yet unborn, not accomplishing goals long sought after. It means leaving behind those for whom life has created joy and meaning. For me to have the opportunity to save a life threatened by cancer or improve the quality of life of someone who is hurting has been my mission since I became a physician. I have cared about my patients and I have grieved and sometimes wept openly when they were hurting or if their cancer was progressing. I truly felt their pain. I have always been committed to helping my patients to the extent humanly possible.

The Talmud, the book of Jewish law says: "Whoever saves one life saves the world entire." This was engraved in a ring made from gold fillings by Jews saved from concentration camps and given to Oskar Schindler of *Schindler's List* fame. This quotation means that even one person can make a difference in making the world a safer and better place. And that was my goal as a physician.

Oncology is a humbling specialty. One must be willing to accept defeat to become an oncologist. As a valued treatment goal, it is necessary to accept improvement in quality of life and, if possible, prolongation of life when cure is not possible. Many of my patients have died. I have mourned for all of them. Many of my patients have survived when that was not the likely outcome given the nature of their disease. I have been thrilled for them and for the loved ones who share their world. I can say with confidence that I did my best for every patient without any motivation for personal gain. I have cared for hundreds of women without insurance and without any expectation of being paid. I think my patients know I was and am committed to them. I think that is why they have so often shared their respect and love for me over the years. The stories that follow concern a few of the lives I have touched over my career. The women in these stories represent just a tiny portion of all my patients that have also touched me as deeply as is humanly possible.

Some have done well in the face of almost insurmountable odds. Others received the best I had to offer and didn't survive. I believe that all knew that I treated them honorably and honestly. I offered no false hopes, yet I always tried to provide respectful and caring treatment. Every name is fictional, changed for privacy. But, to the extent I can recall the details of the diseases and their management, every story is true. Let me share some of these stories and some of life's lessons I have learned by caring for these brave women...

CHAPTER FOUR

SOMETIMES YOU GET LUCKY
KATIE

Katie is a Kiwi. She lives in New Zealand where she was born, but she travels to California frequently to visit her married son and her grandchildren. Katie and her husband were childhood sweethearts. He had a career as a successful professional until his retirement in 2020. He and Katie spent several years in California, a relocation related to his work, prior to her referral to me for care. Katie has always been committed to physical fitness and works out at the gym regularly. She has been a dedicated cyclist, sometimes riding 60 to 70 miles per day. She never smoked, always used sunscreen when outdoors, always went to the doctor for Pap smears, underwent yearly mammograms and had regular checkups. She was pretty much the picture of health.

Katie developed some intestinal complaints as she was planning to fly from New Zealand to California for her son's upcoming wedding in early 2005. She was seen by different physicians in New Zealand and underwent a colonoscopy, a vaginal ultrasound, and had some blood tests performed. Just as she was ready to go to California, she learned from her doctors that there was a pelvic mass putting pressure on the colon. This was thought to be likely causing her intestinal symptoms. A cancer marker, CA-125, on a blood test was abnormal. Normal was less than 35. Katie's was over 1500. Days before her trip, New Zealand doctors told her she likely had ovarian cancer. She could hardly believe it. She had always done everything she was told to ensure good health. She and her husband were understandably panicked. She was able to gain referral to me within a few days of arriving in California.

When I met Katie and her husband, I was so impressed by their devotion to each other and to their family. They are genuinely special people who were well informed of the prior test results and probable diagnosis. My examination confirmed the strong suspicion of cancer, and I recommended that she undergo surgery to confirm the diagnosis of a probable ovarian cancer and to try to remove it as soon as possible. They shared an understanding of my urgency for the operation which I performed just a few days later. The surgery date coincided with their 33rd wedding anniversary and was just two weeks before their son's planned wedding.

At surgery, the cancer was quite advanced as is typical for most women with ovarian cancer. There was spread from the ovaries to the uterus, colon, omentum and several other areas within the abdomen and pelvis. I was able to remove all the visible cancer by performing a complete hysterectomy with removal of the uterus, ovaries and tubes. I also removed the omentum which is a fatty apron of tissue attached to the colon and stomach. The omentum is the most common site of spread from these cancers outside the pelvic organs. And I had to remove a portion of the colon. Fortunately, I was able to reconnect the colon, avoiding the need for a colostomy. I removed other areas of cancer carefully wherever I saw them. This included removing varying sizes of "implants" or growths over the colon and the small intestine as well as other abdominal areas.

Katie did remarkably well and was discharged from the hospital in a few days. However, she developed an infection in the incision that required attention provided by her husband for several weeks before the wound finally closed completely. In a wistful autobiography that Katie shared with me years later, she wrote about her experience following surgery. She expressed doubt that she would "ever gaze at a newborn who would be my grandchild." while she was looking at newborns in the neonatal unit at Long Beach Memorial Hospital where she had undergone her operation.

Two weeks following her operation she attended her son's wedding in a wheelchair decorated brightly by friends for the occasion. When the music of the first dance after the wedding ceremony was played, she got out of her wheelchair and danced with her son. She is a remarkable woman. All that physical fitness paid some dividends that evening and during the months that followed.

Even when all the visible cancer is removed with such advanced ovarian cancers the risk of a recurrence is extraordinarily high, 70% or higher. Katie had stage III-B disease and I planned a course of chemotherapy with two very strong chemotherapy drugs typically used in this situation, Carboplatin and Paclitaxel (Taxol). Typically, this is begun three weeks after surgery, but her wound infection necessitated a delay for a few weeks until she was six weeks post-operative. At that time, I began the chemotherapy every three weeks for a total of six treatments. These chemotherapy drugs have most unpleasant side effects, the most odious of which is total hair loss. There is also nausea and vomiting and often extreme constipation. The white blood cells which protect the body against infections often fall to levels that increase the risk of infections. Even mild infections can be very serious in patients undergoing chemotherapy because the body's immune system has been compromised by both the cancer and the chemotherapy drugs.

Red cell counts often fall markedly, resulting in anemia. Katie experienced most of these symptoms, but she was strong, and she was a trooper. Finally, she completed her treatments in summer 2005 and was well enough to return to New Zealand. The plan was to measure her CA-125 levels regularly and frequently in New Zealand as a rise would indicate that the cancer had recurred.

Just imagine the fear that ovarian cancer patients must carry with them daily, knowing that cancer is likely to return and that if it does return, almost no such patients are curable at that point. Those were the thoughts Katie had when in late 2006 her CA-125 began to rise. She was seen by a gynecologic oncologist in New Zealand who recommended restarting chemotherapy with drugs that were different from those that she had received after her operation a year and a half earlier. She contacted me. My thinking was a bit different. I knew that Carboplatin was the most effective drug for her disease and with a fairly long interval during which she was free of cancer, using it a second time was a better choice than the one she was given. I suggested adding a different second drug, Gemcitabine (Gemzar), along with the Carboplatin and excluding the Taxol she had received previously. She had two choices, one from her oncologist in New Zealand and a second from me.

Katie decided to return to California where I could take care of her. She looked the picture of health despite the knowledge that her cancer had recurred. Her short snow-white hair had regrown curlier than before her chemotherapy. She was dismayed about the possibility of baldness once again now that she finally had a full head of hair after losing it all with her first chemotherapy treatments. Again, six treatments which she tolerated a bit better than the first time in 2005 were administered. Fortunately, she didn't lose her hair, so she was certainly grateful for that little blessing. Taxol always causes baldness; however, I had eliminated it from her chemotherapy regimen. The drugs I put her on this time do not typically cause baldness. She finished her chemotherapy in the spring of 2007.

Based on the natural history of these cancers, I was hopeful she would go into remission and remain disease free for several months, maybe a year or two, but fully expecting her cancer to recur during the ensuing couple of years. We had long discussions about this but, as I always tell my patients, everyone is an individual and statistics are based on populations, not individuals. Just because statistics tell us to expect a recurrence, the future is uncertain and any outcome is possible.

I have stayed in touch with Katie from time to time over the ensuing years, even following my retirement in 2018. I emailed Katie Christmas of 2020, nearly 14 years since that last chemotherapy treatment. She lives in New Zealand with her husband who retired recently. He had been by her side before, during and following surgery, caring for her wound infection, by her side for all the chemotherapy treatments, sharing the fears and uncertainty of her life and giving her the love he always has given her for what now, at that special time of the year, is a happy 49-year marriage. She has remained cancer free. This was not the expected outcome but a welcome one. When she comes to California she visits with her son, his wife and children, and her grandchildren whom she doubted that she would ever see. And she comes in for a checkup, just to be sure she is o.k., and she is.

Sometimes when playing baseball, you think you might be lucky to get a single when the pitcher is out of your league and you are badly overmatched. Then, somehow, you hit a home run. Not too often, mind you, but often enough to make the possibility exciting. This was an unexpected home run against the most difficult of opponents. I like baseball metaphors and use them frequently.

There have been a lot of Katie stories over the years, but not enough, of course, not nearly enough. This outcome was not the result of some special intuition I had. It was frankly just a lot of good luck. I hope you loved hearing about Katie as I enjoy sharing her story. She is very special to me and to a lot of other people as well.

CHAPTER FIVE

ALL'S WELL THAT ENDS WELL

Connie

Most cancer survivors come to believe that their doctors were singly responsible for their fortunate outcome. In reality, for most such patients who survive, other cancer doctors would have achieved the same outcome. In other words, whether I was the doctor, or another gynecologic oncologist was the doctor, the patient would be expected to do equally well most of the time. In fact, in many cases even doctors without specialized training in cancer care would likely achieve the same good result. Among the gynecologic cancers this is especially true for most women with uterine cancers. A straightforward "simple" hysterectomy done abdominally, vaginally, with the laparoscope or with robotic assistance would achieve success measured as "cure" with most uterine cancers, no matter who is the operating physician. This favorable outcome occurs because uterine cancers usually present early in the course of the disease with abnormal bleeding, spread to other organs infrequently, and usually are removed entirely with removal of the uterus along with the ovaries and fallopian tubes.

It turns out that the most frequent of the gynecologic cancers are uterine and therefore are curable in most instances by whomever manages the patient. At the other end of the spectrum of uterine cancers, however, some are very aggressive. They might have metastasized to other organs when first diagnosed and therefore would likely not be curable. Again, this observation is independent of the operating physician. Such patients would likely do poorly even if managed by the most skilled gynecologic cancer surgeon. I should mention, however, that in terms of quality of life and even duration of survival for such women, a highly skilled and well-trained gynecologic oncologist often provides a better result for these unfortunate women even when cure is not the outcome.

But there are some women with uterine cancers whose disease is more aggressive and yet curable, but only in the hands of the experienced gynecologic oncologist. For such patients, the surgical procedure performed is typically more complex than a simple hysterectomy and often requires removal of lymph nodes to which the cancer might spread or nearby organs affected by the cancer. Post-operative management with chemotherapy, radiation, or both can be the difference between survival and death. Often it is not clear which patients with uterine cancers fall into this high-risk category requiring more advanced surgery or post operative "adjuvant therapy" with radiation therapy and/or chemotherapy until surgery is being performed or until the pathological findings following surgery are known. Therefore, it is generally best for all women with uterine cancers to be cared for by a gynecologic oncologist.

Let me introduce Connie, again a pseudonym. Connie was about 45 years old and hospitalized at a community hospital in Whittier, California in May 1998. Her doctor requested a consultation by my partner, Dr. Matt Kohler, who was then and still is an amazing gynecologic oncologist.

Matt joined our group at the UCI Medical Center four years earlier after completing his gynecologic oncology fellowship at Duke University Medical Center. We knew he was a gifted surgeon and researcher. and we were delighted when we attracted him to our institution. Matt and I shared in the care of many patients and often had the opportunity to operate together at hospitals where we didn't have fellows, such as Fountain Valley Regional Medical Center and Whittier Presbyterian Hospital. I digress, but should mention that Connie was one of Matt's last patients before he moved to be with his wife and two children who had moved eastward from California for their own medical issues. Matt currently is a leader in our field at the Medical University of South Carolina, teaching residents and medical students and managing the care of some of the most complicated of gynecologic cancer patients there.

Connie had been admitted to the hospital with a bowel obstruction and was found to have a huge abdominal mass, approximately the size of a full-term pregnancy. The mass was the cause of the intestinal obstruction, and she was unable to eat. As a result, she had lost 25 or 30 lbs. and was "skin and bones," as my mom would have said. She was so unstable on her feet because of her weakness, and the mass in her abdomen that she was mostly immobile. Because she was bed ridden, she had developed infected bed sores. The infected sores caused a blood infection. and she was being treated with strong antibiotics. Additionally, the mass in the abdomen was blocking the drainage of urine from the kidneys, so she was also in kidney failure. When Matt evaluated her, he decided that once she was a bit more stable, gained some weight and was no longer infected, he would operate to remove the mass which he believed to be in her uterus. It was unclear if this was a cancer, but that was his strong suspicion.

Connie was placed on intravenous nutritional support called TPN (total parenteral nutrition) since she was unable to nourish herself otherwise because of the intestinal obstruction. Tubes were placed into the kidneys through her back (percutaneous nephrostomies) to permit drainage of urine and relieve her kidney obstruction. Her bed sores were treated aggressively by her nurses and her antibiotics were continued until she could be operated on safely. Matt took her to surgery in late May and carried out an exploratory operation. He told me afterwards that the mass was in the uterus and every attempt he made to approach its removal resulted in heavy bleeding. He did not feel that the mass could be removed safely. He obtained a biopsy of the mass and closed the abdomen. A few days later he learned that the biopsy revealed a low-grade sarcoma of the uterus. Such cancers frequently can be cured with surgery; however, because of the risk of life-threatening bleeding and serious injury to critically important nerves and blood vessels in the abdomen and pelvis, this did not seem to be the case for Connie. At that point Matt asked me to look after her as he was literally packing his bags and, on his way eastward.

I met Connie a few days later. She was recovering from the operation Matt had performed, understandably depressed, but still hopeful. She was still very thin, had her nephrostomy tubes in her back draining clear urine, was on her TPN and was still on antibiotics. She introduced me to her boyfriend of many years who was devoted to her. Both were resigned to the probability of her dying without ever leaving the hospital. They told me that they wanted to get married before she died. That was her one wish, and of course, I really had no issue with their plans as it had no bearing on any decision I would make. I was now responsible for her care. They did follow through and contacted their clergyman who married them in the hospital room. The ceremony was attended by a few close friends and relatives. Some of her nurses were in attendance. This was quite a story that made the local newspaper. They were somewhat of celebrities, briefly.

I told them I would like to try some chemotherapy in the hope of reducing the size of the mass so it might be removable. The newlyweds both agreed. I started her on a course of chemotherapy typically employed for uterine sarcomas. The probability of a good response was low, but I really didn't feel that I had many options given Matt's findings at surgery. Over the next six weeks Connie was administered two courses of chemotherapy which did absolutely nothing to the mass. It was now causing increasing pain. Accordingly, I decided that if they were willing to assume the risk, I would operate again to see if I could have better success than Matt had. Connie and her husband were grateful that I was willing to try and, with considerable trepidation, I scheduled her for surgery on June 17, 1998. I anticipated that there might be massive bleeding from the tumor so I requested that a vascular surgeon assist me in case we needed to do some heroic vascular procedure to control the bleeding I might encounter. I was assured that the chairman of vascular surgery would be my assistant.

Surgery was scheduled at 7:30 a.m. I arrived just after 7:00. I greeted Connie and her husband in the preoperative holding area and checked to be certain that six units of blood were available for the procedure (a unit of blood is approximately one pint). I also checked to be sure that more blood could be made available if needed. I rechecked her blood studies to be sure that there were no unanticipated issues that would interfere with the operation or her recovery. (For example, a low platelet count caused by the chemotherapy would preclude safe performance of such a dangerous operation.) I didn't see the vascular surgeon, whom I didn't know, but I figured I would meet him in the surgical scrub area. Surprise of surprises, he was not there and was "available if needed." My assistant was a gynecologist and not one who was used to dealing with difficult surgical procedures or management of intraoperative bleeding issues.

The operation proceeded as otherwise planned, with no vascular surgeon, no Matt Kohler who was now back east, and no well-trained fellow accustomed to operating with me on difficult cases. There were just a gynecologist as an assistant and me. I made a large midline abdominal incision from the pubic area up to the xiphoid process at the highest point in the abdomen. I exposed the mass and saw the suture material Matt had used to control the bleeding encountered during the operation he had performed eight or ten weeks earlier. The mass was indeed very bloody (we use the term vascular), but I was able to move it slightly without stirring up too much bleeding. I was able to determine that the area likely to provide the greatest problem was in the left side of the pelvis and that the right side was much freer. Accordingly, I started working on the right side.

As I always taught my residents and fellows, "do what is easiest first." The right side was definitely easier to approach early in the procedure than the left. Once I was able to control the huge blood vessels feeding the tumor in the right side of the pelvis, which I was able to visualize with some difficulty, I went to the left side where everything, including the left ureter, lower colon and rectum, the corner of the bladder, pelvic nerves and blood vessels, were stuck together. I could feel the tube in the left kidney and was able to trace it down into the pelvis. It was obvious that the mass was stuck over the ureter through which I could feel the ureteral stent that had been placed by interventional radiology. A stent is a tube placed in the ureter to keep it open so the kidney on the side of the stent is not injured by a blocked ureter. By placing the stent, not only was the kidney protected, but it enabled me to feel the ureter and therefore avoid injuring it while trying to remove the uterine mass.

In order to approach this area, I was able to systematically control bleeding sources from the left ovary and then the uterus itself. I had to carefully remove the mass that was almost fixed onto the left common iliac artery which ultimately provides blood supply to the thigh, leg and foot on that side. Protecting that artery was critical to the safe removal of the uterus. This went pretty smoothly and finally I had freed up the uterine mass entirely.

The rest was a piece of cake. I sutured the necessary vessels that were supplying blood to the enlarged uterus deep in the pelvis, sutured the supporting ligaments holding the uterus in place and removed the uterus in its entirety. I felt really good. The mass was out and Connie was stable. I completed the operation and went into the waiting room to share the news with her husband. He could not believe it and frankly, I was a bit surprised that the surgery went so well.

The rest of the story is pretty humdrum. Her hospital course was uncomplicated and straightforward. There was no more infection, so the antibiotics were stopped. There was no further need for the nephrostomy tubes or ureteral stents since the mass which had caused the blockage was gone, so they were removed. She was eating like a teenage boy on a track team, so there was no more need for TPN. She went home a few days later with her new husband. There was much fanfare from her nursing staff, as you might expect.

A year later, Connie sent me a personal note. I share its content verbatim here to help understand why what I do is so meaningful for me and so important to my patients and their families:

> Dear Dr. Berman,
>
> This day, June 17, 1999, marks the one-year anniversary of the day, forever etched in my memory, when you performed the miracle of miracles, and saved my life. I cannot even begin to imagine or comprehend what it must have been like for you to be faced with the monumental challenge and task to do what others had said could not be done.
>
> I had been told that the tumor could not be removed, that I would not live much longer, that "there is no hope." I was also told, however, that you are

a brilliant surgeon, the best in your field, and that if anyone could save my life, it would be you.

I remember laying on the operating table, looking toward the foot of the table where you stood. I tried to speak your name. I wanted to thank you then for all your efforts in case there wouldn't be an opportunity later, but I couldn't find my voice. So, I said a prayer for you, placed my destiny in your hands and felt my world slip away. Then, in the fog, I was dimly aware of a shadowy figure leaning down toward me and I heard the words, "the tumor is out" and again, my world slipped away.

It wasn't until I awoke in intensive care and realized that many hours had gone by, that I began to wonder about it all. I wondered about the degree of difficulty with which you were faced. I wondered how long it had taken. I was sorry for all I had put you through. I knew it could not have been easy for you. I wondered where you were, if you felt the enormity of your accomplishment all at once or if it was something that sinks in over time. I lay there listening to the breathing machine behind me and wondered if you were awake or asleep. I wondered about so many things.

Dr. Berman, I can't even begin to find the words to thank you for all you have done for me. I agonize incessantly, trying to decide what I should do to thank you. But anything, everything that I think of pales by comparison How does one thank another for having saved one's life? There is no greater accomplishment on this earth than to save a life. Yet, I know that I owe you my life. Please know that I will always stand at the ready to do whatever I am able to do for you. If you ever need to call on me to help you in any way, I will be there for you, just as you were there for me.

How I wish I could tell you that you saved the life of someone special, but I am quite ordinary with no claim to fame. It is not even so much for myself that I thank you, but for my family. For, even as ordinary as I am, I am one of their loved ones, and because of me, they suffered immeasurably. A suffering that only you could and did dispel. I thank you so much for that. I thank you for the joy you have brought back to them, which brings so much joy to me.

We speak of you daily, thank God for you, give praise to your name. You have no idea you are the standard by which all others are measured. No one stands above you. You are truly a miracle worker, brilliant in your work and beautiful in your person.

Dr. Berman, though my words be wholly inadequate, please know that they are heartfelt when I say, thank you so much for you and for all that you have done for me and for all that you have done to restore my family.

Remembering you this anniversary day,

Forever your devotee and ever so sincerely,

Connie

I believe that Connie is still alive and well. My last contact with her was six or eight years ago, at least a dozen years after her operation. She had continued to do well, without recurrence of her low-grade uterine sarcoma. She kindly gifted the division of gynecologic oncology about $16,000 over three years for our research programs as a thank you to me. That money was put to good use in supporting some of our clinical trials.

In times when I was saddened over the years for loss of a patient or questioning myself whether there was something more that I could have done for a given patient, I have often thought back to June 17, 1998 when Connie and I had quite an adventure together, and that memory always gives me a lift.

In medicine as in life, all is well that ends well, even when a good outcome is not the expected one. There is no moral to this story nor even a special message I would like to share, just a happy ending to a hard day's work for a lovely lady and her family.

CHAPTER SIX

BRCA GENES : JOSIE

Many patients with ovarian cancers I have cared for over the years have had a gene that placed them at high risk for developing this devastating disease. Up to 20% or more of women with this cancer are predisposed to develop it because of mutations in one of two genes that are supposed to protect against developing the disease. These two genes, BRCA-1 and BRCA-2 when normal, or "wild type," are called tumor suppressor genes. That is, they suppress the changes in cells which might become cancerous by repairing DNA damage which occurs naturally. Failure of suppressor genes to do their job can lead to certain cancers which can result from that DNA damage in cells. These two genes normally reduce the risk of breast and ovarian cancers and in fact are named for their protective effect for breast cancers (BReast CAncer gene); however, when one of these genes is altered or "mutated," it no longer has that protective effect.

One of my patients, Gloria, had a mutated BRCA-2 gene, although her medical providers did not know that during her lifetime. I am certain of that because, when her daughter, Melissa, developed breast cancer at the age of 47, she was tested and found to have the mutated BRCA-2 gene. The surviving husband (father) was tested and was negative, so her mutated gene must have come from her mother

Gloria. That accounts for Gloria having developed breast cancer several years prior to Melissa. Gloria's breast cancer diagnosis was made while she was post-menopausal, about 60 years old. In contrast to Gloria, many breast and ovarian cancers caused by BRCA mutations occur in premenopausal women, such as Melissa. In any case, Gloria must have had the BRCA mutation and, we discovered, passed it onto each of her four daughters. Statistically, that was unlikely since the field of genetics would predict that about half of Gloria's offspring would inherit the mutated gene. Remember, however, that statistics predict events among populations of people much more accurately than for individuals. So, in fact, each daughter had a 50% chance of inheriting the gene from Gloria. The likelihood that all four daughters would inherit the gene was 50% times 4, or one in 16. These were low odds, however, that is precisely what happened. Just to put it into perspective, if Gloria had had 1000 daughters—I know that is ridiculous to consider—we know that close to half of them would have inherited the BRCA mutated gene and half would not. A population of 1000 individuals is much more predictable of a disease occurrence or a treatment outcome than only four individuals. A little bit of statistics for the morning (or afternoon or evening, or whenever you are reading this).

Because the mutated BRCA genes place a woman at extremely high risk for ovarian and breast cancers, women known to have the mutation must choose whether to have removal of the organs at risk before a cancer develops or to undergo close observation to reduce the risk of a cancer developing and progressing to an advanced stage even before it is diagnosed. That is especially concerning for ovarian cancers because there is no effective way to detect these cancers before they have spread to other parts of the body. Because of this observation, most women who know that they harbor a mutated BRCA gene will electively undergo removal of the ovaries and fallopian tubes (we now know that many of these cancers start in the fallopian tubes rather than in the ovaries) following completion of childbearing. The decision for management of the breasts is more complicated because many women feel less feminine if their breasts are removed prophylactically than when their pelvic organs are removed. Furthermore, breast cancers usually can be detected at an early stage while curable if evaluated frequently with breast exams, mammograms, and MRI tests of the breasts. Accordingly, many women do not elect to have prophylactic removal of the breasts even when they are at high risk for cancer based on the presence of a mutated BRCA gene.

That brings me to Josie who was BRCA-1 positive and did not know it until she was tested for the gene mutation after she was found to have an ovarian cancer. Josie was in her 40's, married to a loving husband with two biological daughters. Josie presented to her doctors at Cedar Sinai Medical Center with a swollen abdomen and abdominal discomfort. She underwent the usual testing which included a physical examination which showed a mass in the abdomen. An abdominal/pelvic ultrasound showed the mass arising from one of the ovaries and/or fallopian tubes. There was also a lot of fluid in the abdomen, called ascites. Ascites is commonly found in women with ovarian cancers and results from the production of fluid from the cancer itself. A series of blood tests showed an elevated CA-125 of several thousand. Josie underwent a surgical procedure by the gynecologic oncology team at Cedar Sinai Medical Center which was similar to the operation I had performed on Katie and described several pages ago. Josie's cancer was stage III which is the most common stage of disease for this cancer.

Stage 1 cancers, which are confined to one or both ovaries, occur in about 20-25% of patients. Most of these early-stage patients are curable. Unfortunately, this early stage is seen in such a small minority of ovarian cancer patients and did not include Josie. She was treated with the same chemotherapy drugs Katie had received. She did well for a year or two until her cancer recurred in the abdomen and pelvic region. She continued under the care of her doctors receiving additional chemotherapy treatments over the next couple of years, each time after a cancer recurrence was documented. Her care was exemplary. She did as well as patients typically do with this disease.

Josie and her family moved to Orange County, California, and she came to see me as a new patient. When I first saw her, she had obvious disease in the abdomen. She was symptomatic with abdominal pain and she was short of breath. I ordered an abdominal CT scan that showed several areas of obvious cancer. As she was symptomatic and had already recurred following many different chemotherapy regimens, I offered her surgery to try and relieve her symptoms.

I had no expectation of curing Josie. She understood that. I did take her to surgery within a few weeks of meeting her and was able to remove most but not all of her cancer. I tried a new chemotherapy drug that she had not received previously with the hope of prolonging her life. She did remarkably well for about three years at which time she developed a blockage of the colon. With such a blockage she lost several pounds as she was unable to eat and experienced severe abdominal pain. I recommended performing a colostomy so she could begin eating again and to relieve her pain. Without the colostomy, I explained, she would best be placed in hospice for terminal care. She was not ready to die, so she agreed. I performed her colostomy without complication. She went home from the hospital in a few days and lived another three or four months until her death. A team of palliative care physicians handled pain management and general supportive care including psychosocial support for Josie and her family. Her quality of life up until her final days was fair to good.

Shortly after Josie died, one of her daughters who was also BRCA positive came to see me. I had met her previously when caring for her mom. We spent an hour or more discussing her cancer risks. She was in her early 30's, had two children and wanted a third. Her initial concern was breast cancer and she elected to undergo a prophylactic double mastectomy before planning to become pregnant again. She reasoned that she did not need her breasts; however, she certainly needed an intact reproductive tract to have another biological child. I continued to see her for the next four years during which time she had her third child, a girl. She considered her options when her third daughter was about a year old and decided to undergo a prophylactic hysterectomy and bilateral removal of the ovaries and tubes. I performed this operation vaginally at Long Beach Memorial Hospital without complication. She went home the day following her operation. She has done well, lives a normal life, and keeps in touch with me from time to time on Facebook. Her father is happily remarried but was recently diagnosed with pancreatic cancer. Good luck doesn't seem to follow this family, unfortunately!

Josie was loved and is missed by her friends and her family, but her outcome was typical for this disease. I miss Josie, and I think of her often. She understood her disease remarkably well. She knew she was going to die from her cancer when I first met her and began to care for her, but she wanted to live as long as possible if she could do so on her own terms. Throughout the entire time I took care of Josie, she was in control and actively participated in all the decisions about her care. I think that the active participation of patients with cancers and other serious diseases in the decision-making process is so important to their psychological well-being. She was willing to undergo surgery and chemotherapy so long as there was a reasonable expectation of longer survival with a reasonably good quality of life.

I think she and I were able to accomplish that goal. As is true of all my patients, or at least almost all of them, she was very special to me.

The takeaway message here is to emphasize the importance of genetic consultation and testing in women with ovarian cancers and pre-menopausal women with breast cancers. If testing is positive for a BRCA mutation, then testing their family members, who comprise the high-risk population for BRCA associated cancers, is essential. If family members test positive for the BRCA mutation, they must be offered counselling about their risks for breast and ovarian cancers, as well. They should be encouraged to undergo prophylactic removal of the ovaries, fallopian tubes and possibly the uterus after completion of childbearing. Careful screening for breast cancers with frequent mammograms and MRI scans of the breasts or prophylactic removal of both breasts should be discussed with genetic counselors. Whatever decision such a woman makes should be supported by her health care provider while continuing to offer careful monitoring for disease.

CHAPTER SEVEN

GRATITUDE : ZAHRA

There are few gifts more appreciated and powerful than gratitude. When gratitude is directed towards another, both the giver and the recipient benefit immeasurably. Just look back at Connie's gratitude towards me for the care I provided her when her cancer was thought to be incurable, and I was able to remove it for her. I know that she felt so special in sending her thoughts of appreciation to me, while I can't begin to tell you how many times I have thought about her and her graciousness. It has lifted me up and reached the core of my being again and again.

Gratitude often is not directed to another person, rather towards God or perhaps to no one or nothing in particular. How many times have I thought how fortunate I have been in my life to have such special children, a wife of nearly 50 years to share my life, eight fabulous grandchildren, a meaningful professional life, a love of other activities including photography, hiking and travel, and, after Marlene's passing, the love of my girlfriend Bonnie.

I am so fortunate and so grateful for so many things. And yet I didn't do enough to express my own gratitude over the years, to Marlene, to Leo Lagasse who trained me, to Phil DiSaia who opened doors for me professionally that probably would not otherwise have occurred. How many times did I give thanks to my parents for raising me, instilling principles of honesty and hard work, the importance of leading a valued life? Certainly not often enough. And then, as time moves on, the opportunity to express gratitude to others passes, like a cloud or a summer shower. Parents and mentors are no longer with me to visit and share experiences. Most importantly, lost is the opportunity to express gratitude to them.

A word about Dr. Phil DiSaia to whom I will always be indebted. At various times Phil was my mentor, my boss and my colleague, and my friend. He was one of the founders of the specialty of gynecologic oncology. In 1973 when I was a second-year resident at Harbor General, I had the opportunity to attend a scientific meeting in Hawaii. I went there and heard two gynecologic oncologists speak, Dick Boronow from the University of Mississippi in Jackson, Mississippi, and Phil DiSaia who was a young faculty member at the University of Southern California at that time. I was blown away by their talks. It was hard for me to believe that gynecologic surgeons could do the things they were doing in the operating room. They talked about bowel resections, bladder reconstruction, plastic surgical procedures, etc. That was the first time I ever considered going into the specialty. I wanted to be able to do those types of operations.

I met Phil again in early meetings of the Society of Gynecologic Oncology in Key Biscayne Florida later in the 1970s He was like a god to me. I didn't really think he knew I existed. He later would write the most frequently used textbook on gynecologic cancer entitled *Clinical Gynecologic Oncology* along with his best friend, Dr William Creasman in 1981 and subsequently a total of ten revised editions over the next 40 years. His book was on the bookshelves of most OB/GYN physicians for two generations! Given his stature in the specialty, I was more than surprised when he contacted me in early 1981, five years after I finished my fellowship training to offer me a job at the University of California, Irvine, as an associate professor. I was Director of Gynecologic Oncology at the University of Pittsburgh at the time. That call changed my life personally and professionally in so many ways when I accepted his offer to move west. Sadly, now deceased, to this day, when people speak of the most important and influential physicians in our specialty, Phil's name is always among the first to be mentioned.

Now more about gratitude: I loved reading the book *Mayo Clinic Guide to Stress Free Living* by Amit Sood. I have read it three times and each time I am gifted with new ideas to improve the quality of my life. I have embraced many of his observations and suggestions in my life and I have incorporated some of them in this book. Many of these concepts are similar to those referred to as "mindfulness," whose origins arose in Buddhist and Hindu teachings and were popularized in the West by the work of Jon-Kabat Zinn, professor emeritus at the University of Massachusetts Medical School. In the "Mayo Clinic Guide to Stress Free Living," Dr. Sood suggests that one practice gratitude daily.

I think that is a great idea. He advises that we awaken and think of those we love and those who give meaning to our lives, and mentally express gratitude towards them. Maybe each of us can direct our positive thoughts to four people that are special to us in any of a thousand ways. Intentionally think of four such individuals each morning and start each day on such a positive note.

Let me share Zahra's story with you. Zahra, which means "flower" in Arabic, is Egyptian. She understands the importance and value of gratitude. Zahra is a social worker. Perhaps by training or just by virtue of her nature as a caring person, she knows how to express gratitude. My first contact with Zahra occurred in 2005 while I was in my car in the doctor's parking lot at Fountain Valley Regional Medical

Center. My cell phone rang and, even though I was on my way into the hospital to see a patient with a newly-diagnosed cancer, I answered the call. I didn't recognize the number, but I usually did answer my phone calls while I was actively caring for patients. Nowadays, with innumerable robocalls daily, and being retired, I no longer answer calls from sources I don't recognize.

Zahra was obviously in a panic mode. Her speech was hesitant and then rapid, speaking between sobs. She had been under the care of a gynecologic oncologist locally in South Orange County, California for a cancer of uncertain origin. Sometimes it is not possible to be certain where a cancer arises; however, it is important to know, if possible, because treatment decisions often are dictated by the origin of the cancer. She told me she was 40 years old and had undergone surgery for what was thought to be a cancer in her uterus. The doctor who performed her operation found that the cancer had spread within the pelvis and that she was treated with chemotherapy after she recovered from surgery.

When she contacted me that afternoon she was feeling well; however, scans and her pelvic exam showed that there was still cancer present. She was told that she was not curable, although there were other treatments that her doctor would like to try. When she heard that she was not curable, she was inconsolable as most 40-year-old people would be. She got my name somehow and wanted another opinion about her options and her prognosis. I told Zahra that I would be happy to see her, review her records and make recommendations to her. She seemed so relieved just to know that I was willing to see her. She thanked me.

I met Zahra, who really is a flower in many ways, early the next week. She is a beautiful person just as a flower is a thing of beauty. She brought all her records with her for my review. After I reviewed the records and had my pathologist review her slides, I suspected that she did not have a uterine cancer after all. I told her I believed that she had a very unusual cancer which arose from endometriosis in the pelvis. I thought this was more hopeful for her. I suggested we consider another operation to see if I could remove all the endometriosis I suspected was present. If I was correct, by removing the endometriosis which contained her cancer, her prognosis might be better than her prior doctor thought.

I had seen several such patients over the years and had successfully treated many of them. Zahra readily agreed. Her operation was scheduled within a couple of weeks. I took her to surgery and found extensive endometriosis as I had expected and I removed all evidence of it. The pathologist subsequently found many areas of cancer in the removed tissue, which I had expected. I also removed her lymph nodes in the pelvis, some of which also contained cancer. At the end of the operation there was no remaining visible cancer; however, I knew that Zahra's cancer was at high risk to recur. Accordingly, after she had recovered from surgery, approximately one a month later, I had her see the radiotherapist who agreed that a course of radiation might reduce the risk of her cancer recurring. The radiation was delivered over six weeks. Zahra tolerated it remarkably well. Her operation was in April 2005 a few days after her 40th birthday and her radiation was completed that summer.

On April 5, 2010, Zahra sent me an email. The subject line read "Dr. Berman I am 45 years old today!"

She wrote:

> I just wanted to share with you how happy I am. Today is my birthday and I am just so happy and grateful to be here and doing well. I celebrated with my family yesterday and after my mom finished thanking God...she thanked you. Dr. Berman you take care of me as if I am your only patient. You know exactly the right kind of balance of kindness, humor and bluntness to use with me... I just want you to know, that whatever happens

in the future, I feel blessed. I wish I could say that I was certain that I would celebrate my 45th birthday five years ago when I was diagnosed but I was not, until you became my doctor. With much gratitude!! Zahra

Zahra keeps in touch with me by email. Here is another note she sent me in 2017.

Hi Dr. Berman,

My birthday was yesterday, turned 52 and had a great time! I hope you never get tired of me telling you how much I appreciate how much you have done for me to ensure that I continue to have quality to my life and celebrate another year. My appreciation grows more every year, if that is even possible. When I work with clients as a Social Worker, I try to always relay the same compassion that you have shown me and my family. I can truly say I am a better Social Worker for having gone through this journey and having you as my doctor.

Very truly gratefully,

Zahra

I continued to see Zahra in my office at Saddleback Medical Center until my retirement in June 2018. She is doing well and sends me a note every April. She wanted to purchase one of my photographs since she knows that I am a photographer. I turned her onto my web page and she liked several of the images, but she asked for my suggestion. I recommended "Storm Brewing" but suggested that in her case it would be renamed "Storm Passed," for surely her storm has passed and she is cured. The photograph on the cover of this book is the one Zahra selected. I chose the book title, "Storms Passing," because the stories I am sharing are of women who came to me during their personal storms, the most frightening storms of their lives, and for whom the storm was passing or had passed. Zahra tells me she loves the image and remembers me whenever she looks at it. And of course, I remember Zahra every April and throughout the year.

CHAPTER EIGHT

FORGIVENESS : KARISHMA

Forgiveness of another is one of the most difficult acts for most of us. It certainly has been for me at times. Yet I know just how important it is to remove the negativity that anger towards another person creates. I mentioned "The Mayo Clinic Guide to Stress Free Living" before. I really like what Dr. Sood had to say about forgiveness. "So, what is forgiveness? Forgiveness is a choice that you make to give up anger and resentment, while acknowledging that misconduct happened. Forgiveness is choosing a higher path. Forgiveness is for you, not for the forgiven. Forgiveness is your gift to others, even those who are undeserving of your kindness."

Let me share a story about forgiveness I dealt with several years ago. It is a personal story and difficult one for me to tell because it brings back negative memories. I try to avoid negativity and embrace positive thinking to the extent possible in my life.

Many years ago, I was angered and hurt by the actions and words of two colleagues whom I had considered to be friends. It seemed to me that they were collaborating to harm me professionally. They spread lies about my care of patients and my interactions with trainees. Their words seemed to be believable to some colleagues and it adversely impacted my professional interactions with them. It even carried over to my personal life and at times I avoided social gatherings because of fear of rejection by friends.

I would find myself ruminating about these two colleagues, sometimes when I was trying to get to sleep, or taking care of patients, or when I was with my family, or even away on vacation. My anger could arise anytime, anyplace and under any circumstance. I really could not escape my hatred of what they had done to me for several years even though their allegations had been proven false and they had moved on to other positions elsewhere. It was still affecting the quality of my life.

Finally, one day, I was on a treadmill at a 24-Hour Fitness center in La Brea, California again thinking about these two former colleagues. I came to the realization that it was critical for me to get past this anger, not so much for them but for me. I resolved to forgive them as soon as I got off the treadmill. I kept running and walking for another hour so I could get out all the anger I held inside. And when I got off the treadmill, I forgave them and never again focused on their actions. By no means did my forgiveness validate their actions which were reprehensible, but I felt better instantly. It was as if I had lifted a weight off my chest. When I left the gym, the air felt fresher, the sky seemed bluer, and my tired muscles felt more relaxed. I felt free and frankly joyful. I have never reignited my anger towards them. Mahatma Gandhi and Dr. Martin Luther King best stated attributes of those who can forgive: "The weak can never forgive. Forgiveness is the attribute of the strong" Gandhi. "Hate can't drive out hate; only love can do that." Martin Luther King.

So, with that background, let me share another patient whom we will call Karishma which means "miracle" in Hindi. Karishma was not of

Indian origin or heritage, but her story is a miraculous one. Karishma was 25 years old when I first met her in 1993, and she had recently undergone a cesarean section with delivery of a term pregnancy. At the time of her cesarean section a mass was found on an ovary. A biopsy diagnosed "Small Cell Carcinoma" of the ovary. I had never seen a patient with this diagnosis. Small cell cancers arise more commonly in other organs such as the lungs, uterus, cervix, etc., but rarely in the ovary. When I reviewed the medical literature, I was dismayed to see that for this exceedingly rare cancer no one had ever reported curing such a patient. I carried out an exploratory operation in 1993 and found widespread cancer staged as III C. I performed a complete hysterectomy with removal of the ovaries and tubes, removal of the omentum and removal of all the visible cancer in numerous locations throughout the abdomen and pelvis.

As no one had ever cured such a patient, to my knowledge, I didn't see much value in administering the usual chemotherapy drugs typically used for ovarian cancers. Rather I decided that if we were to have a chance at longer survival than typical for the disease or even a possible cure, it would require a novel and very aggressive approach. I explained all of this to Karishma, who was agreeable to try anything. She was a new mom. Most moms will do almost anything to be around while their children are growing up.

I devised a chemotherapy regimen using six different drugs that best targeted small cell cancers and ovarian cancers respectively. I was careful to select drugs wherein the toxicity between them did not overlap excessively. I didn't want to cause her death before the cancer would be able to do so. She was young and otherwise healthy, so I thought she would be able to tolerate the six-drug cocktail better than someone older. Furthermore, there was little to lose, since we anticipated an early death with conventional therapy. In the medical literature, most of these patients died in less than a year.

Frankly, there was no reason to expect that she would do well even with this combination of drugs; however, my course of treatment was borne out of desperation.

Remarkably, Karishma tolerated the six courses of treatment without excessive toxicity. She did lose her hair, experienced severe nausea and vomiting, and had severe reduction of her white blood cells. Her platelets were also severely depleted which placed her at increased risk for hemorrhage and infection; however, she did not bleed, she did not get infected, and she survived her treatments. Four years later she had remained free of cancer. This was significant as there had been no women who had survived so long. I was ecstatic and encouraged my fellow at the time, Dr. Krish Tewari, to write her up as a case report so other such patients under the care of other physicians might also benefit from our experience with this complex drug regimen. Krish published the case report in October 1997.

The following year I received a notice of intent to sue from an attorney representing Karishma. While administering chemotherapy in 1993, I had inserted a portacath into her chest. This was typical in such circumstances to facilitate the safe administration of the chemotherapy drugs through large veins in the chest. Unfortunately, a small portion of the portacath had eroded through the skin of her chest and caused her local discomfort, so she was suing me for it. I was stunned and initially did not know exactly what to do. And then I decided to send the attorney a copy of the case report that had been published. She was identified in the case report by her initials. The report indicated that she was the only reported survivor of advanced small cell ovarian cancer in the world. She had no detectable cancer during the follow-up period because of the novel treatment she had received. I sent the report to the attorney with the following four-word cryptic note attached to it: "This is your client." And I signed it. That was the last I heard from the attorney and, for that matter, the last I heard from my patient. I am hopeful that she is alive and well, but I am glad that she was not enriched through payment for her "suffering" from her portacath.

Karishma was so fortunate. To my mind, her action in seeking out an attorney was reprehensible. Yet I was happy for her that she lived long enough to recover and try to find a way to help support herself as she raised her child. I do not think I was ever very angry with her; however, I forgave her and continue to wish her well.

As a postscript, I received a note of thanks in December 2001 from another patient who lived in Buffalo at the time. She was 22 years old and was recently diagnosed with small cell carcinoma of the ovary. Her doctor had contacted me after reading the case report written by Dr. Tewari and asked for my advice about her treatment. I provided the chemotherapy regimen to her doctor that he was using to treat her as well. She was grateful for giving her hope while facing this terrible disease. I only wish her well but do not know if she survived this tragic disease. It remains among the rarest and deadliest of all cancers.

CHAPTER NINE

EMPATHY AND COMPASSION
JILL AND MEGAN

Are empathy and compassion the same emotion? That is an important question. They are related but not the same. Empathy is the ability to sense, to relate to, and even to feel the emotions of another. Compassion is a higher goal, to react to the emotions of another with the goal of helping that individual. It is easy to be empathetic but requires effort to be compassionate. Empathy is passive, compassion is active. Both are measures of concern for the well-being of others and both are of value. Compassion is practicing the Golden Rule of treating others as you want to be treated. All of us should feel empathy for our fellows but how often do we act on that feeling. Who is not empathetic for people without enough to eat but how often do we give our time or our money to make a difference in the lives of people in need?

Importantly, compassion enhances the well-being and happiness of both the giver and the receiver. Yet there should be no expectation of reward or even acknowledgement for being compassionate. In fact, expectation of reward contaminates compassion. The best place to start exhibiting compassion is in your own home by being less judgmental and being more accepting of family members. Random acts of kindness are beautiful expressions of compassion. It is also important to be compassionate to oneself. All of us are imperfect and deserve the right to comfort ourselves. Just think about that for a moment. We actually deserve self-comforting.

Perhaps we can assume that physicians are compassionate by nature. Having made the choice to help others as one's life's work illustrates compassion and selflessness. Lawyers or engineers or plumbers or electricians certainly can be empathetic and demonstrate compassion, but it is not a requirement for the job. On the other hand, it is a requirement for a physician, or at least it should be. We deal with patients who are their most vulnerable and in greater need for compassion than at any other times in their lives. Interestingly medical school applicants are evaluated by their interviewers for this trait; however, there is no precise or reproducible way to measure a sense of empathy or a commitment to performing compassionate acts in most individuals. Sure, if an applicant has done a lot of charitable work in college, this gives a powerful hint of things to come as a physician; however, there are lots of physicians who simply are not terribly empathetic or charitable towards their patients. I know this is true, partly based on my own observations of physicians' practice patterns over the nearly 50 years of my career, and partly from so many complaints from patients about seemingly insensitive doctors who have cared for them in the past.

Many physicians perceived to be less sensitive than the job should require might have been more empathetic in the early years of clinical practice following completion of their training; however, changes in medicine over the past 25 years have removed much joy from the practice of medicine for many which might have changed their perspectives on patient care. Physicians often have endured loss of control of their practices when taken over by managed care organizations or hospital entities. They have experienced reduction of their income by federal legislation and the need for competitive contracting with payers. They object to the increasing malpractice exposure in a litigious society, and the expenses they incur to protect themselves from possible litigation. They often order unnecessary tests for their patients as a defense to possible malpractice claims and then they are blamed for the increasing costs of medical care. There are substantially increased practice expenses required to accommodate the requirements of governmental and insurance regulations and yet there is no additional reimbursement to cover those increased costs.

These real-life changes in the practice of medicine undoubtedly affect how a physician might view his or her career choice, and therefore his approach to delivering medical care. Lost is the opportunity to sit and chat with a patient about their concerns because financial constraints require that a physician be efficient in the practice of medicine. Efficiency does not allow for chatting. Patients may be viewed as adversaries, at times, rather than partners in their care. It is an unusual physician who enjoys fighting with insurers to obtain authorization for needed tests for a patient or for an indicated procedure. And yet, that scenario is all too frequent in the lives of physicians and their staff. It is possible to become desensitized to the joy of performing compassionate acts when surrounded by so much negativity.

More physicians retire early in their careers than ever before and even suicide is increasing among physicians. "Physicians die by suicide at twice the rate of everyone else," reads an article in the *Washington Post* in October 2020. I believe these observations reflect, in part, the draconian changes in the practice of medicine that have occurred during the years I was an actively practicing gynecologic oncologist. And yet, physicians are still highly respected for the dedication they demonstrate and the work that they do to ease suffering in their patients. And I still believe that choosing to be a physician is a higher calling for an individual, a choice to give a higher purpose and meaning to one's life. The opportunity to perform compassionate acts for thousands of patients is truly a blessing.

Let me apologize for that rant about insensitive physicians and adverse changes in the practice of medicine and get back onto the target of compassionate care. I believe the care I administered to my patients *was* compassionate and caring. That was always my goal. Yet, there have been occasions wherein I have had the opportunity do more than provide good care, to make a difference in the lives of my patients and their families, beyond the scope of the direct care I provide to my patient. It is a little like Christmas or Hanukkah in which I come bearing gifts for the whole family rather than just my patient. You might think of it as winning the exacta in a horse race by betting on the first two horses in their order of finish and winning on both. Or you might think of hitting a home run to put your team ahead in the top of the 9th inning and then saving the game with an amazing catch in the bottom half of the inning. Such opportunities are welcome but not common.

Now, let me tell you about my patient, Jill, and her daughter, Megan, to illustrate how a compassionate act can at times enrich a family.

Jill came to see me in 2012 as most of my patients do, by referral from her physician. I do not recall if it was her family physician who found a lump in her umbilicus or her gynecologist who found a mass in her pelvic region. Suffice it to say that Jill, who was accompanied by her husband of 27 years, had a malignant process arising in the pelvis. When I saw Jill, she was tearful and apprehensive. She had noted a discoloration in her umbilicus (often called the "belly button") that had bled on a few occasions. She had gained weight, but her face looked thinner than normal. Her abdomen was swollen.

My examination confirmed the lump, or what we call a nodule, in place of her umbilicus. Her swollen abdomen had obvious fluid in it, and I could also feel a mass. A CA-125 cancer marker was elevated, and I was confident that she had stage IV ovarian cancer. Cancer growing through the umbilicus would qualify as stage IV.

I counseled Jill and her husband about the likely diagnosis and the need for surgery followed by chemotherapy. At that same visit I came to learn that they had a daughter, Megan, who was interested in becoming a physician. She was in the process of applying to medical schools. I didn't meet her at that time. Jill was anxious to undergo surgery which was scheduled in about a week.

Indeed, at surgery I found what I had expected, an advanced ovarian cancer with extensive involvement of her omentum in the upper abdomen. The omentum had attached to the abdominal wall at the level of the umbilicus and had grown right through the umbilicus. This has a name, a Sister Mary Joseph nodule. Sister Mary Joseph was a nurse who became William J. Mayo's first surgical assistant from 1890 to 1915. William was one of the famous Mayo brothers who founded the Mayo Clinic many years later. Sister Mary Joseph was an extraordinarily skilled nurse who first drew attention to the nodule in a patient with a cancer arising in the abdomen. These growths occur most commonly in patients with ovarian, gastric, colonic, and pancreatic cancers. Dr. Mayo published the finding which subsequently has carried the name of his nurse.

Surprisingly, there was not a lot of cancer present in Jill other than in the ovaries and the omentum. In order to remove all the cancer, I had to remove her umbilicus along with the omentum as well as perform a complete hysterectomy (uterus, ovaries and tubes). It would have been easy to close the abdomen after removal of these organs, but I wanted to give her a new umbilicus, since people expect to have one of them. They are used to looking down at their abdomen and seeing a "button," something to break up the landscape down there. It could be an innie or an outie, but a button was expected to be there. (In case you are interested, it is a lot easier to create an innie than an outie and, frankly, innies are prized much more than outies, so that was my plan.) So, I fashioned an umbilicus by puckering the skin in the area where the umbilicus that I had removed should have been. Then I sutured the wrinkled-appearing skin to the underlying supporting tissue of the abdominal wall. It looked beautiful, just like a belly button and, more importantly, the entire cancer had been removed.

Jill had an uneventful post-operative course and was discharged in a few days. Three weeks later I started her on the usual chemotherapy regimen of Carboplatin and Taxol for six cycles at three-week intervals. Her CA-125 was now normal and her examination was normal as well. Although she had stage IV disease by virtue of cancer growing onto the abdominal wall, I was optimistic about her chances of cure since I had easily removed all the visible cancer. I began seeing her every three months after completion of chemotherapy and her exams remained normal. Unfortunately, the umbilicus that I fashioned for her no longer looked like a typical umbilicus. It had become just a flat area of scar tissue in the middle of her abdomen. I was a bit disappointed; however, she told me she didn't mind at all.

Two years later, in September 2014, I was invited to speak as a guest professor at my alma mater, George Washington University School of Medicine, during Homecoming week. The presentation was the annual Allen Weingold lectureship. The lecture series is funded from an endowment by Dr. Oscar and Mildred Dodek.

In 1937, this Dr. Oscar Dodek founded the Kane King Dodek Obstetrical Honor Society at George Washington University. His nephew was also named Dr. Oscar Dodek who later chaired the Department of Obstetrics and Gynecology at George Washington University. In 2014 Dr. Nancy Gaba was Department chair. She succeeded Dr. Dodek. Dr. Dodek had succeeded Dr. Allen Wiengold, the conference's namesake.

First side note: Along with Dr. Herb Kotz. the younger Dr. Oscar Dodek was my wife's (Marlene), obstetrician when we were living in Washington, DC. Drs Dodek and Kotz delivered three of our four daughters, Mara, Lisa, and Debbie. You might want to read the dramatic details of my daughter Vicki's delivery several years later in Long Beach California, during my residency at Harbot UCLA Medical Center as told in my autobiography.

Second side note: Dr. Weingold, in whose name my lecture was given, was my sister-in-law Lorraine's obstetrician when she was pregnant with her third child, Lindsey. He performed Lorraine's tubal ligation following the delivery. Normally a tubal ligation is a simple procedure with a low risk of complications; however, in this instance it was complicated by hemorrhage the day following the procedure. The resulting blood loss required numerous blood transfusions and resulted in her becoming infected with Hepatitis C, a serious and often life-threatening liver infection. I think this unexpected complication helps to remind me that all procedures have risks, and one must always weigh the risks versus the benefits of any surgical procedure.

Dr. Dodek (Marlene's Obstetrician) was in the audience during my talk which was entitled "Strategies for Stress Prevention." I learned later that Dr. Dodek died in 2017. I always considered him a Renaissance man with his amazing intellect and curious mind. He graduated law school after obtaining his medical degree at George Washington. And he was the first Board Certified Reproductive Endocrinologist in the Washington, DC area where he went on to establish the Department of Reproductive Endocrinology at George

Washington University Hospital in 1978. He was actively involved in Human Rights and Women's Health issues. And he was known for his generous philanthropy.

Dr. Dodek's partner, Dr. Herb Kotz, was ill or I am certain he would have attended the lecture as he and I had become close friends over the years. Herb was fellowship-trained in Gynecologic Oncology at the MD Anderson Cancer Center and was a respected cancer specialist in the DC area. Herb was very involved with research activities at the National Institutes of Health (NIH) while also working at George Washington and was honored by the creation of the Herb Kotz Award given annually to the outstanding fellow in oncology at NIH. Without success, Herb had tried to recruit me to George Washington to lead their Gynecologic Oncology program. I was saddened to learn that he died a few months after my lecture.

My lecture was remarkably well-received and afterwards I entertained questions from the audience. A psychiatric attending physician said she was sure I had put my talk together with help from the Department of Psychiatry since it was hard for her to believe that someone outside of the field of psychiatry would have such insight into stress prevention. (I didn't have any help, by the way).

After my lecture ended and the audience began to disperse, a young attractive blond woman came up to greet me shyly. She was Megan, Jill's daughter. She wanted be certain that I was her mom's doctor and then to thank me for caring for her mom. She was a freshman medical student and came to the lecture because she thought I might be the physician caring for her mother. I chatted with her for a while, and she told me that she was interested in becoming a dermatologist after graduating from George Washington. I was delighted to meet Jill since I didn't know that she was successful in getting into medical school and certainly had no idea that she was at my alma mater.

I shared my meeting Megan with Jill on her next visit; however, she was already quite aware of it. Jill's husband even brought in a George Washington University baseball cap for me to take home. Interestingly, I do not think George Washington has a baseball team, but they do sell baseball caps.

Over the next couple of years until my retirement as I continued to follow Jill, who was doing fabulously well, I learned that Megan was applying for a residency in dermatology at several hospitals including UCI. It appeared that UCI was her first choice, especially since her mother's outcome was uncertain and she wanted to be near her mom. I spoke with a few of the folks I know in the Dermatology Department about Jill and her daughter, Megan, and shared her story with them. If nothing else, at least those calls to other faculty made Megan's name known to them when she applied for residency in the department. In any case she was accepted into the highly competitive dermatology program at UC Irvine Medical Center and currently is a second-year resident. Obviously, I have no knowledge whether she was selected, in part, because of my input; however, it certainly didn't hurt her chances at all! And Jill, now eight years following surgery and chemotherapy, remains perfectly healthy and cancer free. Jill sends me a Christmas card each year and updates me on her continued disease-free status and shares information about her family. And, from time to time, I wear my George Washington University Medical School baseball cap and I am reminded of Jill and Megan.

CHAPTER TEN

LUCK
ADRIENNE, EVA AND OCTAVIA

Shifting gears a bit, I was thinking about how luck can sometimes be a game changer in medicine as in life. Sometimes it is good luck, sometimes it is bad luck, and sometimes it's a little of both. I know that I have benefited from a great deal of good luck over the years. I recognize it and am grateful for it. Sometimes luck is just being in the right place at the right time. I often think back to when I was offered a fellowship by the faculty at UCLA while I was a resident on rotation at the City of Hope during my third year of training. The stars just came together while on that rotation (that is a poetic description of luck). I had decided that I didn't want to be awakened in the middle of the night as an obstetrician anymore or practice office gynecology, but I had not decided how I wanted my career to move forward. I loved surgery and had the perfect rotation at the City of Hope with an abundance of cancer patients needing surgery, chemotherapy or end of life care. The rotation opened the exciting world of complex abdominal and pelvic surgery to me at just the time when I was feeling pressure to make a career decision.

The gynecologic oncology fellow from UCLA who was on rotation at the City of Hope during my clinical rotation there was a good physician and a very nice person but not terribly assertive. His failure to take over management of the gynecologic oncology service or to establish ground rules for our respective roles in the operating room gave me the chance to shine while he largely remained in the shadows. He should have taken the opportunity to demonstrate his clinical skills to the UCLA faculty there, but I was more aggressive than he was. He allowed me to function largely as the fellow for the three months I was there and I took advantage of the opportunity.

Another bit of good luck was my timing in considering a career as a gynecologic oncologist, because when I began my training program in 1974 there was little to no competition for fellowship training in gynecologic oncology. The specialty was so new that it was not on the radar screen of many obstetrical residents. When I was a medical student from 1963 to 1967, there was no such thing as a gynecologic oncologist. The first organizational meeting of physicians who wanted to establish a specialty of gynecologic oncology occurred in January 1969 when I was in my first year of residency. The first scientific meeting of the Society of Gynecologic Oncologists was held in 1970 just after my arrival in Alaska with the Public Health Service. There were only 57 members of the Society in 1970 in the United States. Even by 1979, three years after I completed my fellowship, there were only 147 members throughout the country. So, I considered myself lucky to be among a select group of physicians when I obtained a fellowship from 1974 to 1976.

Fellowship training programs in about 25 institutions had just been established with training guidelines in 1972. Examinations to prove competency in the specialty were just being developed while I was still a resident. To add to my luck, when considering doing a fellowship, I balked at the offer of a fellowship position initially because I hesitated asking Marlene to live for another two years on the salary of a trainee while raising four young Berman children.

I was rewarded for my hesitation with the offer of a faculty position as Acting Assistant Professor with a salary that accompanied that position.

And then after completing my fellowship I really did not know what I wanted to do with my new skills, but my mentor, Dr. Leo Lagasse, one of the finest physicians I have ever known, invited me to stay at UCLA where I could refine my clinical abilities. So again, timing was right for me as the UCLA obstetrics and gynecology program was in a growth phase and had an opening for another faculty position. So , I stayed on as an Assistant Professor for a year until 1977. I gained a great deal of confidence that year, taking care of my own patients yet with experienced colleagues around should I need any assistance or wish to discuss a complicated patient with a more senior colleague.

Around that time, in 1977, the specialty of Gynecologic Oncology was first being recognized as important to academic programs around the country. I was contacted by Dr. Terry Hayashi, the chairman of the Department of Obstetrics and Gynecology at the University of Pittsburgh, Magee Women's Hospital. This was one of the largest and most respected hospitals for women's health in the country. I was not looking for a new position at the time and was quite happy at UCLA; however, I was in the right place at UCLA at the right time. I was offered the opportunity to build a gynecologic cancer program at a prestigious women's hospital just one year following completion of my training. It was a great opportunity which I accepted. I had a productive four-year experience in Pittsburg between 1977 and 1981. The program grew under my leadership and I even recruited a new colleague to my gynecologic oncology division, Dr. Harrison Ball, who had trained at the University of Pennsylvania. I was happy with my career and Pittsburgh was an exciting city, especially for a sports fan like me. The Pirates won the '79 World Series and the Steelers won the '79 and '80 Super Bowls which I attended.

But Marlene was unhappy, and she thought that she was destined to live out her days in a city that she really did not like at all.

As mentioned, I was not even considering leaving Pittsburgh, frankly despite Marlene's unhappiness and worsening rheumatoid arthritis. And again, I was in the right place at the right time. I took that call from Dr. DiSaia who offered me the position at the UC Irvine Medical Center as an Associate Professor with tenure. That offer occurred in the spring of 1981. The faculty position I was offered guaranteed me an academic position there for as long as I chose to stay. It promised the opportunity to train residents and fellows, earn a handsome income, return to the place that Marlene and I loved most (maybe tied with Alaska), enjoy the fabulous Southern California climate, and live happily ever after. Well, of course, people do not live happily ever after, because like the stock market, there are ups and downs. Still, life was good, and our return to Southern California was very lucky rather than the result of something I had actively pursued.

I think the stars have always been aligned for me. As I have said so many times, I have never actually looked for a job, and yet I have had numerous fabulous positions over a 50-year career, lots of it the result of incredibly good fortune. I have lived long, and I have lived well, surrounded by people that I love and who care for me in return. I have made a great difference in the lives of many people and I have been rewarded with their kindness and gratitude. Life has truly been good to me, but I know that luck had a lot to do with it.

So, let me tell you about Adrienne as I share a story about good luck. Her medical history is not so extraordinary, but she illustrates how luck can make a great difference in our lives. Adrienne was sent to me with a huge mass on her vulva (the external genital region) in the fall of 2005. She was 92 years old at the time. Older women often tend to be very modest about their personal privacy and try to avoid examination of their genital area by a physician. Adrienne had noticed a lump for at least a year but was hesitant to have it examined. When it became painful and began to bleed, she felt she had no choice. She went to see a physician who took a biopsy which confirmed the clinical impression of a vulvar cancer. Her doctor sent her to me for further evaluation and management.

Typically, when I was still in practice and had a new patient, I would review the demographic information she provided to my nurse before I first met her. This information usually included her occupation in addition to date of birth, marital status, address, next of kin, insurance, etc. For this particular woman, I was especially interested in her occupation which was listed as director of a speech and language development center. This special-needs center had opened its doors about 50 years earlier, and Adrienne had been its director since its inception. I came to learn that it had a great reputation locally and nationally and had received substantial federal and state funding for its special-needs programs. My grandson, Tyler, who is my daughter Vicki's son, had been diagnosed as autistic just a few months earlier at two years old, so I was very interested in what she could tell me about her center and the services they provided.

I told her about Tyler. She expressed a great deal of interest in him. I suspect she was more comfortable talking about him than she was about her newly diagnosed cancer. In any case, after speaking together for about 15 minutes, I had her taken to the examination room where I confirmed her cancer diagnosis and outlined a plan of surgical management.

Adrienne's surgery went well despite her advanced age. The surgery is typically very extensive and wound breakdown is quite common; however, she healed perfectly and was discharged just a couple of days following her operation. When she came back to see me in the office about two weeks later, my first question to her was "How are you doing?" and her first question to me was "How is Tyler?" That began a relationship that led to Tyler's being admitted to her Speech and Language Development Center for speech and language therapy, occupational therapy and physical therapy beginning in February 2006. This continued until he was three years old. He made some real advances during the eight or nine months at the facility.

His special-needs program that was developed there for him continued as he transitioned to the public school system beginning with preschool in 2007. One thing I learned as Tyler has grown and matured is that early intervention is critical to the development of autistic children. Adrienne provided that for Tyler by giving him such an important head start in life following his diagnosis. He is now a third-year student at the University of Nevada with excellent grades and plans to become an attorney.

I continued to follow Adrienne for five years until she was 97, still cancer free but now wheelchair bound because of arthritic changes in her hips and knees. Every visit for the five years of follow up would begin with "How is Tyler?" She had finally given over the reins of the center she had nurtured and loved for more than half a century to her very capable daughter who continues to run it to this day. I lost track of Adrienne after she was 97 years old, but I will always be indebted to her for her caring attention to Tyler and the difference she made in his life, Vicki's life, and mine.

I would be remiss if I didn't point out that lady luck lives on a two-way street. One side is "good" luck and the other "bad." Sometimes it is unclear which side of the street one is walking or driving on. For example, if you miss your plane, it seems like you are on the bad luck side of the street; however, if you learn later that the plane crashed, you realize you were on the good luck side. On the other hand, sometimes your perceived good luck is actually just the opposite.

The Washington Senators had a pretty good pitcher named Tom Cheney. On September 12, 1962 he pitched the game of his career against the Baltimore Orioles. In that game he threw 228 pitches over 16 innings and struck out 21 batters, a major league record to this date. These days pitchers almost never throw more than 110 pitches in a game. In any case, he set a record that has not been matched in nearly 60 years; however, the damage to his shoulder caused by this one masterful game virtually ended his career. He didn't pitch again that year and although he did win eight games the following year. His career was essentially over by the age of 29.

I might also mention that Lady Luck Avenue meets a cross street called Promote Luck Way. Doesn't it seem that certain people have all the luck? Some people just seem to have good things happen to them and for them. They are the ones who just happen to get the good grades in school, get into the prestigious colleges and graduate schools, get the great jobs, make lots of money, marry the perfect partner (sometimes), have just the best home and the best kids. How do some people have all that luck? Hmmm. Maybe some of them live on Promote Luck Way where the locals there just seem to do the right things that somehow result in good luck. They study hard in school, they take direction from their mentors, they seek out friends who understand the distinction between right and wrong, they exhibit honesty, they assume responsibility for their actions, they follow the "golden rule," they are upstanding citizens, and then somehow, they just get lucky. Thomas Jefferson once said, "I find that the harder I work, the more luck I seem to have." I am just saying, it's probably all just dumb luck.

So, let me show how fickle lady luck can be by telling you about one of my Pittsburgh patients, Eva. I first met Eva in 1978 when she was referred to me with abnormal uterine bleeding. She was in her late 30s at the time and an elementary school teacher. She underwent a D and C (dilatation and curettage) to obtain tissue from the lining of the uterus. This showed an unusual cancer called a stromal sarcoma. Whereas most kinds of uterine cancers are highly curable, those with the designation of "sarcoma" can be very aggressive. Stromal sarcomas often are advanced when diagnosed. Even when they appear to be confined to the uterus they can recur in other parts of the body after a hysterectomy and can cause death. At least 30 to 40% of women with stromal sarcomas die of their disease, and of those who are cured, almost all of them have disease that is apparently confined to the uterus when diagnosed.

I carried out surgery on Eva and, unfortunately, found that the cancer had spread to the lower abdomen and pelvis. Even though removal of areas where the cancer has spread for this type of cancer rarely results in a cure, I did remove the areas of spread that I could identify. Still, I knew that the probability of a cancer recurrence for Eva was extraordinarily high, at least 90%, so I recommended further treatment.

In the 1970s the only treatment of sarcomas that had any benefit was a drug called Adriamycin or Doxorubicin. At times the drug has been given the nickname of "red devil" because of its color and its side effects. Besides the common side effects of hair loss, nausea, vomiting, infections, anemia and mouth sores, Adriamycin can, at times, cause irreversible heart damage. Heaven forbid that a few drops of the drug gets into the tissues of the hand or arm while it is being injected intravenously as it will cause deep third degree burns and extensive tissue damage that will not heal. Despite these side effects, this is a very valuable drug and is commonly used in the treatment of breast cancer patients, and patients with various types of sarcomas, as was the case with Eva. It's also effective in treatment of some of the childhood malignancies.

I was not optimistic that Eva would do well but was pleasantly surprised when she remained free of cancer for the next three years before I left Pittsburgh to take my new position at UCI. I lost track of Eva after that until I received a note from her dated Sept 17, 1992, which was 14 years following her operation and chemotherapy. She had seen an article in *Good Housekeeping* listing me among the 400 best cancer doctors in America and she wanted to reach out to me to let me know that she was thinking about me and that she was still alive.

As her note read:

> "I've had no recurrences of any cancer and I'm so thankful you were in Pittsburgh at the right time." She noted, "However, in 1986 I had a virus that affected my heart and did very well until last fall. I have idiopathic cardiomyopathy and was put on the list for a transplant (heart transplant) in April. I'm feeling good though and teaching half-time..."

It is not possible to say whether the need for a heart transplant was from the virus, or the Adriamycin or perhaps a combination of the two. What I can say is that the drug likely contributed to her improbable cancer cure but might have damaged her heart such that she would require a heart transplant many years later. I do not know if she had a heart transplant or how she has done since that nice note in 1992. Lady luck is an unpredictable lover, but all of us continue to pray that she will look on us with kindness.

I have one other story about luck that came to mind while I was deciding what I wanted to share about Adrienne and Eva. I will call this patient Octavia since this name comes from the number eight and this story is about numbers. I do not recall very much about Octavia. I cannot see her face when I think about her as I can do with many of the patients I am sharing in this book. She was one of so many patients I cared for many years ago. This was probably between 2000 and 2010. I do remember she had an advanced cancer, probably ovarian and that things did not go very well for her. She did not live a long life following her diagnosis, maybe a year, perhaps two years. I do recall that she was young with two or maybe three young children and a husband who was devoted to her. I recall that her surgery was not as successful as most and that she did not experience the good response, although often temporary, that most women with ovarian cancers will have. Her story was a tragic one as so many of them can be. And then, as the end approached, arrangements were made for terminal care and comfort measures. These last acts of care are so important to patients and to their families. They provide for a time, although brief, in which goodbyes can be said and wishes expressed. Her only wish that I recall was that the family stay together and that her husband and children should have a good life. And then she was gone.

Her husband came by to thank me for my care of his wife a couple of weeks later. We sat and talked for a half hour or more. He told me about his difficulty in coming to grips with the loss of his wife, the mother of his children. And then he told me a story that still resonates when I consider how fickle life can be. He shared that for the years they were married, they always loved playing the lottery and did so daily. They had picked their numbers early on, probably related to birth dates or home addresses, or whatever moves people to select certain numbers for the lottery. They had always played the same six numbers.

The day Octavia died, her husband was so distraught that when he drove by the convenience store where he usually bought his tickets, he thought he would just drive home to be with his kids. But instead he stopped, played the same six numbers which undoubtedly made him feel close to his now departed wife and then he went home. I had a strange feeling as he told me this story as you, the reader, probably do as well, because you know what is coming next.

He hit the lottery with an eight-figure payout, assuring that he and his children would be okay financially in the years to come. A statistically improbable event; however, you have to wonder, you just have to wonder. Does lady luck actually have a heart, or perhaps a great sense of humor, or is luck always just the result of statistical probabilities? Afterall, someone must win the lottery. It is not always the neediest or most deserving. That is for sure. In any case, I could not have been happier for this family during their difficult days following their tragic loss, softened just a bit by a measure of good luck.

CHAPTER ELEVEN

PERSEVERANCE
CANDY AND TINA

Now let me mention perseverance in the context of surgical care because it can be the difference between a favorable outcome and an unfavorable one. Understandably, Webster's definition is much broader than a surgical context and describes perseverance as "continued effort to achieve something despite difficulties, failure or opposition." So, perseverance can be the continued pursuit of a love interest or learning to tie fishing flies until you get it right, or batting baseballs from a ball machine for hours each day as my neighbor, Shawn Green, did for years before he became a professional baseball player for the Toronto Blue Jays and then the Los Angeles Dodgers. It can be a child learning the alphabet or a chef trying to recall the ingredients in a recipe. But here we are addressing the perseverance that can offer a woman cure of an advanced cancer or prolong her life even when cure is not a likely outcome.

I should also note that perseverance has a twin named *focus*. You never find perseverance without focus, although most of the time focus does not need perseverance nearby. You can be focused on a painting or one of my fabulous photographs, or a flower or a child at play; however, none of these actions require perseverance. Focus is incredibly important in life. When the brain is focused on a task the brain becomes engaged in that task. Dr. Sood from the Mayo Clinic observed that the brain considers the object of focus as interesting, novel and meaningful. The brain can become so engaged that outside distractions might not even register.

Many times, in the operating room I was unaware of what was going on around me while I was focused on a surgical procedure. According to Dr. Sood, focus is a purposeful and a positive action controlled by a high cerebral function as distinguished from what has been called the default mode of attention in which the mind is wandering. In the default mode, the mind is on autopilot or spontaneous thoughts are jumping around without identifiable purpose.

Unfortunately, this default mode in which the mind wanders and is easily distracted, typically visits unresolved issues or personal flaws and, at times, creates an unhappy state of mind. Whenever I have a difficult time falling asleep, I find that my mind wanders from thoughts about the events of the day and plans for tomorrow to unpleasant issues that are unresolved in my life. In other words, my mind is not focused and is in the default mode with thoughts that meander and prevent me from falling asleep. Goals of stress management emphasize the importance of teaching the brain to focus intentionally throughout the day to enhance joy and creativity. Paying more attention to focused thought results in a concurrent reduction of time in the default mode of attention. Simply stated, a focused brain creates happiness and positivity whereas the default mode creates negativity.

There are few places in medicine where perseverance accompanied by focus is more critical than when a surgeon is operating on an unusually complicated or advanced surgical problem. The problem does not have to be a cancer; however, many advanced cancers, especially ovarian cancers in the field of gynecologic oncology, by their nature, require perseverance and focus if the goal is complete and safe removal of the cancer. That is not to suggest, however, that all advanced cancers should be removed completely, even though the need to remove all of the cancer when feasible might seem intuitive. For example, if a patient has an advanced cancer of the pancreas or liver or lung, there is no particular benefit of removing areas to which the cancer has spread. Such a surgical effort does not increase the likelihood of cure or prolong life but does add to the risks of complications for these cancers. But for the gynecologic cancers, especially those arising in the ovaries and uterus, complete removal of the cancer is incredibly important in maximizing the chances for cure.

I know I was often cited at UCI for my focus and perseverance in attacking the cancers that affected my patients. I always wore that badge of honor with pride. One of my graduating residents, Doctor C. Terence Lee, put his thoughts to paper regarding my surgical approach to cancer management on the occasion of his graduation from the residency in June 1994. I enjoyed the poem:

> It's puzzling to imagine and quite hard to determine
> How anyone could operate as well as Michael Berman.
> When he steps into the OR in his surgical attire,
> And he reaches for the bovie and the surgiclip applier,
> No tumor can escape his hand, no adhesions can prevent him
> From taking out the lymph nodes and removing the omentum.
> We all recall as interns, the expressions on our faces
> As we watched him work his magic in achieving hemostasis.
> He taught us how to tie our knots and cauterize so well
> That we could do a TAH(Hysterectomy) with just 50 EBL.
> Someday perhaps we'll grow to be as skilled as he would like
> As they say in that commercial, "If I could be like Mike."

Terry went on to do a fellowship in reproductive endocrinology and is in practice of infertility management in North Orange County. I haven't seen him since his graduation but greatly appreciate his tribute memorializing his perception of my surgical skills. What he is describing is the importance of perseverance, focus, and hard work in the operating room when I am taking care of one of my patients while also teaching residents and fellows how to operate.

So, now I would like to introduce Candy who is a Jehovah's Witness. From a medical perspective, this means that she would not accept blood under any circumstances, even to help manage life-threatening bleeding. This is a Christian religion that follows many tenets unique to their Christian beliefs. The one that affects surgeons, such as me, is their opposition to blood transfusions because of the scriptural admonition against the "consumption" of blood (Leviticus 3:17). Over the years I have operated on dozens if not a hundred or more Jehovah's Witness patients who were sent to me because of my reputation for not losing much blood when I operate. I was always happy to take care of these women. I didn't seek them out; however, the local leaders of their faith would recommend their referral to me, and I was always respectful of their religious beliefs. I always told my Jehovah's Witness patients that I would never give them blood or blood products unless permitted to do so. I also told them that if bleeding became excessive, I might need to perform a lesser operation than I would otherwise do rather than have them bleed to death. Looking back over my career, fortunately I never had to compromise the surgical procedure since none of them had life threatening bleeding that was uncontrollable. I did have a few who had a great deal of blood loss, but I never gave blood as I had promised not to do so, and all of them survived their operations.

Candy who was 34 years old came to see me upon referral by her obstetrician. She had presented at 23 weeks of pregnancy with heavy vaginal bleeding. Her examination revealed a large cervical tumor which was biopsied and proved to be a cervical cancer. When she was sent to me, she was anemic, a common result of heavy or prolonged blood loss. She very much wanted to carry the pregnancy until the fetus was viable. If she were not pregnant her best option would have been radiation therapy with chemotherapy which likely would have been curative; however, the radiation therapy would kill the fetus and, therefore, was not an option in this instance. I decided that we might be able to stop the bleeding with packing against the cancer and that we might be able to correct her anemia with intravenous iron injections and a biological agent, erythropoietin, which stimulates the body to make red blood cells much faster than it normally does.

Candy was brought into the hospital and had a vaginal pack placed against the tumor in the cervix. She was put on strict bed rest to minimize the risk of bleeding and was started on iron injections and erythropoietin. Her hemoglobin was about five grams when we started (normal is about 12 to 14.5). Over the next 11 weeks we were able to raise her hemoglobin to normal levels and, fortunately, she didn't have episodes of hemorrhage, which would have been disastrous. Finally, when tests showed that the fetus was mature enough and would survive delivery at about 34 weeks (7.5 months) we decided to do a cesarean section to deliver the infant in addition to a radical hysterectomy with a pelvic lymphadenectomy to treat the cancer. This was a risky undertaking because of the greater probability of operative hemorrhage in pregnancy during a radical hysterectomy than in the non-pregnant woman. The pelvic blood vessels late in pregnancy are three to four times the size of these same vessels in the non-pregnant woman.

I took her to surgery with Dr. Krish Tewari (the same one who wrote the Foreward to this book). The operation went remarkably well.

There was little blood loss, the infant and mother did well, and the cancer was completely removed. This case was unusual enough that Krish subsequently wrote this up as an interesting case report which was published in *Gynecologic Oncology* in 1998. These kinds of cases come along infrequently and when they do, create a great deal of angst among surgeon, patient, and family. This clinical situation with a favorable outcome would not have been possible without the perseverance to manage her aggressively but expectantly for nearly three months in the hospital. It then demanded focus needed to perform a risky lifesaving operation with a high risk of hemorrhage, in a pregnant woman who could not accept blood or blood products. Candy was subsequently lost to follow up so, I do not know her outcome; however, based on statistics for her stage of cancer, the likelihood is that she survived her cancer to raise her child.

I would like to share another exciting case whose surgical management required the greatest degree of perseverance and focus to achieve a good result. Let me introduce Tina, a 55-year-old Vietnamese woman. She presented to her doctor in 2012 with a rapidly enlarging mass in her abdomen. She was undergoing an exploratory operation by one of the Obstetrician Gynecologists at Fountain Valley Regional Medical Center when I received an emergency call to the operating room there. I was at my office at UCI and quickly drove over to the hospital. I called my fellow, Dr. Sara Jordan, to give me a hand since the cryptic information I received by phone suggested a large bloody mass attached to virtually everything in the abdomen and pelvis. Her surgeon would have just closed her abdomen if that could be done safely, but he could not control the bleeding from the tumor. If he had closed the abdomen, she probably would have continued bleeding.

By the time Sara and I arrived, blood was being infused and the surgeon was sitting in a chair anxiously waiting for my arrival. He had done all he felt comfortable doing and was just waiting for me to take over his operation. After changing into my scrub clothes and Sara into hers, we washed at the surgical sink, were gowned and gloved by the scrub tech, and positioned ourselves across from each other at the OR table. I always stand at the patient's right side since I find that is best for a left-handed surgeon. (I do everything left-handed in the operating room and in my day-to-day activities when operating in the pelvis of a patient.) Sara was on the patient's left side.

We removed the surgical packs placed by her Obstetrician Gynecologist to reduce bleeding and we confirmed the presence of a bloody tumor likely arising from an ovary or, perhaps, the uterus. It was not clear which was the case as both ovaries and the uterus were extensively involved with the tumor. I did obtain a biopsy which I sent to the laboratory for a "frozen section" to determine what type of tumor we were dealing with. Later, perhaps 20 or 30 minutes after we sent the specimen to the pathologist, we were told that it looked malignant (a cancer) but the type of cancer was unclear. Knowing the type of cancer when operating in such a situation is very important since the cancer type often can dictate the most appropriate operation in such a circumstance. For example, if this appeared to be a cancer arising elsewhere, such as the stomach, there would be no reason to remove the mass as that effort would not result in a better outcome than just leaving the mass in place. In such an instance, the patient would not do well no matter what operation was performed. In this situation, we proceeded without the knowledge of the type of cancer we were dealing with.

As soon as we took over the operation, we focused on evaluating just what was involved with the tumor. I recall that there was extensive attachment of the tumor to several portions of the small intestine as well as the mesentery of the intestine. The mesentery is what attaches the intestine to surrounding tissues and contains the blood vessels that supply the intestine. If the blood vessels are disrupted, a portion of the intestine might die. When a portion of the bowel is removed, it is typically done along with the mesentery containing that portion of the blood vessels to the bowel. When there is excessive involvement of the entire small intestine, it is not possible to remove all the affected bowel without creating a situation in which the patient will not be able to nourish herself after recovering from her operation. At least a third to one half of the small bowel is needed to permit digestion of nutrients into the body. In contrast, if the large bowel (colon) is extensively involved with cancer, it can be removed entirely, if necessary, because the colon does not aid in digestion of food.

This was one of those cases where I could not safely remove all the affected small bowel mesentery because it was so extensively involved with the cancer, so I carefully removed tumor on the surface of the mesentery wherever that was technically feasible while still protecting the blood vessels feeding the bowel. There were a few areas where it was not possible to preserve the bowel mesentery, so I had to remove those areas of bowel along with its mesentery to prevent the bowel from becoming obstructed by the cancer. Furthermore, my goal was to remove all the visible cancer to offer her the best chance of long-term survival. Then I had to reconnect the small intestine where portions of it had been removed. All the while, everywhere we worked the tumor would bleed and there were no means by which we could completely control the bleeding. At times, the bleeding was severe enough that we had to stop what we were doing, focus and evaluate. We would put pressure packs against the areas that were bleeding to allow the anesthesiologist time to give her more blood to catch up to what we had lost. As soon as he caught up, we would restart the operation. When we got too far behind in blood loss, we would stop and wait for anesthesia to catch up again.

This happened two or three times during the operation.

But we were making headway. First, we removed the tumor in the abdomen and then we approached the pelvis where the tumor appeared to have started. Everything in the pelvis was stuck together. There were no surgical planes we could develop to facilitate removal of the tumor. This means that there was no separation of the organs and tissues in the pelvis. In other words, the normal anatomical relationships between the pelvic organs were markedly distorted.

Now, I will sidetrack for a few moments and tell you all you need to know to be a world class surgeon. There are four laws of surgery that I have taught my fellows and residents throughout my career. They are laws rather than rules because, like most laws, you can get away without obeying them most of the time and still avoid a disaster. For example, you can speed while driving a car and rarely will you get caught by a highway patrolman, or you can file a fraudulent tax return and rarely will you hear from the IRS. Sometimes, however, just as with laws that guide our conduct in life, you get caught breaking the law and then must pay a serious price. That price for a surgeon can be severe hemorrhage, lacerating an organ such as the bladder or liver, cutting a major blood vessel, a nerve, or the ureter, for example.

The four laws are pretty simple to memorize but take a career to master. Most surgeons, never master them. I have taught them to my residents and fellows for decades. Many of them have told me that when they are in trouble in the operating room, they first say to themselves, "what would Dr. Berman do" and then, as they calm down, they recall the *four Berman Laws of Surgery* which they then try to apply to the surgical situation before them.

The four Berman Laws of Surgery

1. You can and should cut through tissues that you can see through.
2. When you are unable to see through tissues you must carefully palpate, or feel through the tissues, before cutting them to avoid injuring a vital structure such as the ureter or the bowel.
3. Very importantly, you must do what is easiest first because what initially appears to be very difficult becomes easier as soon as easier parts of the operation have been completed.
4. And finally, it is not possible to operate safely if the anatomy is distorted (This was the situation with Tina.) Accordingly, it is necessary to restore normal anatomy.

That's it! That's all there is to it! Now even the untrained reader can spay his or her cat or take out his or her grandmother's appendix on the kitchen table. Maybe not, but those are the rules, and when I see that a surgeon has had to call me to get him or her out of trouble, I suspect that the four rules of surgery have not been obeyed.

Now let me go back to the case at hand. Tina was certainly a challenge. The easier avenue would have been to control bleeding with electrocautery, suturing and possible packing against the bleeding areas and then closing the abdomen. This avenue would have left much of the tumor behind and likely would have required a second operation at a later date to remove the packing once all bleeding had stopped. That thought never entered my mind. We worked in the pelvis for a couple of hours, controlling bleeding, restoring normal anatomy, cutting what we could cut safely, doing what was easiest first, and finally we were done. 25 to 30 pints of blood were administered during the procedure and a few more the first 24 hours after surgery, but the tumor was out, and Tina was safe.

Her recovery was slow because removal of multiple portions of the small intestine requires a few days, typically, before a patient can begin nourishing herself. Still, she did remarkably well.

As I had not met Tina prior to surgery, I had the chance to introduce myself as well as my fellow the following day. I met her husband as well. As is so common with patients from Southeast Asia, she was incredibly grateful for performing the operation on her cancer. She said she could not believe that I would come to the operating room to operate on her when I didn't even know her.

Tina's cancer was a Gastrointestinal Stromal Tumor, abbreviated GIST. Even though I had removed the visible cancer in her abdomen and pelvis, based on how extensive it had been, I knew it was destined to recur. I referred her to a medical oncologist and after careful assessment she was started on a biological drug called Gleevac (Imatinib). Gleevac is a potentially lifesaving drug for this type of cancer as well as some types of Leukemias. She did fine for six years and remained disease free during that time. Her Gleevac was never discontinued during this time because recurrences of GIST frequently occur with discontinuation of the drug. When these cancers recur, they can be highly aggressive with a marked acceleration of tumor growth and a rapidly fatal course. I continued to follow Tina every few months for a few years and then every six months after she remained disease free for three years after her operation.

I saw Tina a few months before my retirement, around six years after her surgery. On my examination I found evidence for a recurrence of her cancer. I shared that information with her and her treating medical oncologist who agreed with my findings which were confirmed on a CT scan and an MRI. At that time, she was switched from Gleevac to Sutent (sunitinib) which is another biological agent that is effective but not curative for this disease. Tina continues to do remarkably well and has kept in touch with me on Thanksgiving every year since I retired. She has given me gifts in prior years, which I discourage, but receive graciously. I will reproduce her most recent email message she sent to me in late November 2019.

> Dear Dr. Berman,
>
> Thanksgiving is the time to remember and appreciated (sic) the benefactors who have saved my life.
>
> My husband and I are forever thankful to you for your compassionate heart and skillful hands with superb experience that have saved my life. May God bless you and keep you safe, happy in your retirement.
>
> HAPPY THANKSGIVING!
>
> Sincerely, Tina
>
> P.S. I just would like to quickly update you on my health: From June 29, 2019 to July 6, 2019, I stayed in UCI because the recurrence of GIST. The tumor had come back. The surgeon team said it was unresectable!! However, I am taking Sutent. Sutent is the second line of defense after Gleevec. The tumor size had shrunk 90% after three months of treatment. I am doing well right now. I am in Fort Lauderdale, FL for a wedding of my niece this Thanksgiving. We always miss you and remember you.

I did receive another handwritten note from Tina on Thanksgiving 2020. She continues to do well and she also sent me a personal gift. I hope to hear from her again over the years to come. Perseverance and focus won the day for Sara and me that afternoon in 2012 and Tina and her family are grateful for our efforts. Her immediate survival was completely dependent on the surgical procedure we performed.

CHAPTER TWELVE

A NOTE ON THE PRICE OF CANCER PHARMACEUTICALS

Before I move on to share some of my other stories, I want to talk about the newer targeted therapy drugs used to treat many patients with various types of cancers. Gleevac and Sutent are two of them used in GIST patients and they are game changers for patients with this unique cancer. Gleevac is more commonly used to treat Chronic Myelogenous Leukemia (CML) which is a much more common cancer than GIST. These types of drugs are referred to as targeted therapy or precision medicine or personalized medicine or biological therapy. Biological therapies can stimulate the immune system or attack specific cancer cells by inhibiting cellular function in these cells. Gleevac, for example, inhibits an enzyme (tyrosine kinase) which is made by a specific gene in some cancers such as GIST and CML. This inhibition results in the death of these cancer cells. Targeted therapy has been effective in the treatment of a fraction of patients with specific cancer types including breast, ovary, lung, melanoma, and others. Research is underway to develop more drugs that will benefit more cancer patients and to identify which patients are most likely to respond to therapy with these new agents.

What I would like to discuss is the cost of these drugs alongside their benefits. We call that a cost benefit assessment. Before I begin, I should mention that every new targeted therapy approved from 2014 until 2019 when I looked up the figures quoted below, cost more than $120,000 per year. I think that is a lot of money to treat one patient for one year. As you will see, the pricing of drugs can really get out of hand.

Gleevac has certainly been a game changer for Tina. It appears that Sutent might be as well. These are exciting new drugs; however, they are very expensive. It is important to remind you that there is a limited amount of money for healthcare in this country and elsewhere, so the treating physician should always be aware of costs of care when considering expensive treatments. Now, of course if you happen to be the patient, you likely will not agree with this premise because no amount of money is too much to treat ourselves, especially when someone else is footing the bills.

Any drug that offers a longer life or even a possible cure is worth whatever it costs is what most patients with a serious disease would say. But wait a moment. Suppose that a drug costs $10,000,000 and would extend your life by a year. Would you agree that, at least from the standpoint of the payer, that might be excessive? In fact, how much money is an additional year of life worth. Again, from the perspective of the patient and her family, any amount is fair game. Not so from the standpoint of the payer, whether it is a private insurance company such as Anthem or a federal payer such as Medicare. So again, how much is an additional year of life worth.

It turns out that some countries have come to a decision in this regard. In the United Kingdom, Canada and Australia, an additional year of life is considered to be worth about $50,000. If a treatment costs $55,000, it might get through a review carried out by a payer, but not $10,000,000 or $1,000,000 or $500,000 or even $100,000 for an anticipated additional year of life. Sure, if you have the money you may choose to spend it to cover the cost with your own funds, but do not expect the payer to cover it for you. As all of us should know by now, life is not always fair, and wealth *can* buy happiness, sometimes.

Now, what about the United States, because, after all, that is where many of my readers live. What are the rules that determine how much a payer is responsible for when a life can be prolonged with a new, expensive drug? Well, it turns out that there is no such established threshold in our country. So, as a result, it is left up to the treating doctors to decide how to treat their patients. The payer can object to an exorbitant cost of therapy, but if there is scientific evidence that the proposed drug prolongs life by any length of time, a year, six months, three months, or whatever, the payer is obligated to cover the costs within the contractual details of the patient's insurance policy. If the insurance happens to be Medicare, it will be covered to the extent that Medicare covers costs of drugs for that patient. As an interesting aside, even though the US covers these costs much more generously (or perhaps foolishly) than, say, the United Kingdom, our life expectancy for our cancer patients is not greater than theirs. In fact, our life expectancy is lower than that of many countries that are less generous than ours for chemotherapy coverage, or any manner of healthcare for that matter.

Now, let me talk about these newer targeted therapies to treat cancers. I'm going to mention some numbers, but you don't have to be a mathematician to get the points I will be making. Let me mention Gleevac again briefly. This drug was introduced by Novartis in 2001. The annual cost of the drug was about $26,000 when it first came out. The cost increased yearly by about 15% on average so by 2013 it cost $80,000 per year, by 2014 it cost $132,000 per year, and by 2016 it cost $146,000 per year. It didn't cost any more to for the drug to be manufactured between 2001 and 2016 but those were the charges.

Interestingly, the actual cost to manufacture one year of Gleevac for one patient has been quoted at $159. Now, in defense of Novartis, there are substantial costs in research and development of new drugs. Furthermore, patients and insurers rarely pay the full amount that is listed as the cost of the drugs. Insurers have contracts with Novartis that substantially reduces their costs and patients without insurance are often charged based on need and ability to pay, to a certain degree. It turns out that the patent on Gleevac expired in 2016, so other drug companies can now produce the drug, likely at about $159 per year's administration, and many have done so. As a result, costs have come down a bit, at least for the generic equivalent of Gleevac. In fact, the generic form of Gleevac from Canada came down from $146,000 to $8,800 per year after 2016 and the generic form of the drug manufactured in India came down to $400 per year. The purchase price from India represents a 99.7% reduction in cost as compared with the patented drug in the United States. You can still purchase the patented drug at $146,000 in the United States or at $38,000 in Canada (it is the same drug mind you) but why would you? Probably because patients and doctors sometimes have a bias against generics, without justification in most instances.

So, what about Sutent which Tina was receiving when I last heard from her? It is another fine drug which listed for just under $234,000 per year in the United States in 2019. For no good reason that I can understand, the identical patented drug in Canada cost $65,000 per year. Unlike Gleevac, the patent for Sutent has not expired. Accordingly, it is not possible to purchase a generic form of this drug, because it does not yet exist. I love Tina for her courage and loyalty to her family and to me and she is truly a very special woman; however, really, $234,000 per year of tax dollars (she is a MediCal patient) for one year of extended life? It would not happen in the United Kingdom; however, of course it wouldn't have to happen there because the drug company sells the drug to the UK at a price that is acceptable to them for administration to their citizens.

Let me take this discussion one step further. Gleevac is used most commonly for Chronic Myelogenous Leukemia patients because CML is much more common than GIST. Again, it is a lifesaving drug for this disease and can be dispensed in its generic form for $400 per year if purchased from India. That is like hitting a home run against Clayton Kershaw while using a bat made of cheap plastic. (I am a lifelong Los Angeles Dodger fan and Clayton Kershaw, who pitches for the Dodgers, is the greatest pitcher of his generation.) It just does not seem possible, but it is true. But wait, there are some newer biological agents that have come on the market recently that seem to have fewer side effects. They are no more effective than Gleevac, but patients might feel a bit better. Unfortunately, a cocktail of these newer drugs is very expensive. More unfortunately, doctors are prescribing these newer drugs because they can, and payers must pay for them. As compared with generic Gleevac, which works just as well, this cocktail of drugs cost about $884,000 per year of extended life, as compared with $400 for the generic Gleevac. You can't make this stuff up!

My entire career I have argued that physicians should know what drugs cost and should consider costs when making treatment decisions. I brought this up when I gave lectures, when I attended meetings in which clinical trials of targeted therapies were being developed and when I have met with the members of my own division of gynecologic oncology at UC Irvine Medical Center. My arguments have fallen mainly on deaf ears.

Here is a personal observation that I think is relevant to the discussion of cost versus benefit of expensive therapies. Physicians have lost control of the practice of medicine and yet most do not have a clue how that happened. They don't understand how and why the Federal government and insurers have taken over physician reimbursement or how HMO's and other entities that manage costs have taken over the control of the practice of medicine that physicians enjoyed in the past. Frankly, it is the unwillingness or inability of physicians as a group to control costs that has resulted in these changes. The manner in which we choose to administer drugs to our cancer patients without sufficient attention to costs illustrates this observation. But the failure of medical schools and residency programs to emphasize the importance of considering costs when practicing medicine is the root cause of these changes that have occurred over the past quarter century.

CHAPTER THIRTEEN

DEALING WITH GRIEF
THE FIVE STAGES

Cancer patients can go through the five stages of grief just as people who are facing death do. Being diagnosed with cancer certainly represents a loss to the patient, loss of control, loss of health, and possible loss of life. During a career working with dying patients, Dr. Elizabeth Kübler-Ross first addressed the stages of grief in 1969. They include denial, anger, bargaining, depression and acceptance. Let me address these stages as related to my own observations of some of my patients.

DENIAL. I have seen patients who are in denial when diagnosed, although not often. These women often request second and third opinions, refuse radiation or chemotherapy or surgery when indicated, or just disappear for a while. This can effectively delay needed treatment while they are in denial. It is axiomatic that denial, while dealing with the stress accompanying a new cancer diagnosis, is harmful to the patient when it results in delays in treatment.

I still remember a young woman who came to see me with a newly diagnosed early-stage cervical cancer in the early 1990s. She was in her late 20s, unmarried, and had no children. I counseled her about the treatment options of surgery or radiation therapy and told her she had about an 85% probability of cure for her stage I-B cancer. I recommended surgery since it would allow me to preserve her ovaries and avoid the premature menopause caused by radiation therapy and chemotherapy which was the other option. When she came to understand that both treatment options would render her infertile, she refused any treatment and disappeared. She came back to see me about a year later and was having a lot of bleeding and some pain. She wanted the surgery that I had described to her; however, her cancer had advanced to stage II-B such that surgery was no longer an effective option. On the other hand, radiation therapy combined with chemotherapy offered her a 65 to 70% chance of cure. I made that recommendation. But she was afraid of the side effects of radiation and chemotherapy and especially the loss of ovarian function caused by the radiation which would have induced menopause in her. Again, she refused treatment. She came back to see me about a year later, her symptoms were worsening. She was now ready for chemotherapy and radiation treatments. Unfortunately, imaging showed that the cancer had spread to other parts of the body (stage IV-B), so while radiation treatments would likely control her bleeding and improve her pain, it was no longer a curative option. She wanted an alternative opinion, and never returned to see me.

I knew that she was no longer curable. She likely died within a year or two after that last visit, suffering increasing pain and probably loss of bowel and bladder function. Patients with incurable cervical cancers typically have so much pain in the pelvis and back that they lose interest in eating. Their focus for the remainder of their lives becomes pain control. These unfortunate women lose a great deal of weight, become emaciated and susceptible to infections that, themselves, can cause death. This was likely her outcome. I felt helpless because she was so curable when she presented to me and ultimately died unnecessarily. Denial in the face of a serious diagnosis can have lethal consequences.

ANGER. I have observed that anger is infrequently expressed after a cancer diagnosis, but it does happen. I found that typically a woman who never smoked cigarettes or drank alcohol, who always watched her diet carefully, and worked out regularly may exhibit anger and disbelief if she developed a cancer. I have heard, "Why me? I always have my regular checkups; my Pap smears have always been normal. I don't drink or smoke. How can I have cancer?" And this dialogue is offered with a measure of disbelief and anger.

While regular checkups which includes Pap smears help protect women from developing cervical cancers, unfortunately they offer no protection against developing ovarian cancer or uterine cancer. In fact, regular checkups do not even protect against a woman presenting with an advanced and incurable ovarian cancer, although regular checkups do reduce the risk of being diagnosed with an advanced uterine cancer. Actually, a healthy diet with good weight control and regular exercise does reduce the risk of developing the most common type of uterine cancer. Unfortunately, ovarian cancers are usually not discoverable until they are advanced, even if a woman had exams as often as three or four times a year. I recall a patient who had undergone laparoscopy for infertility at which time her findings, which were confirmed on multiple images taken during the procedure, were normal. Three months later she presented with an advanced ovarian cancer. These silent cancers spread before symptoms or physical findings suggest cancer is present. Interestingly, a history of birth control pill usage is one very effective means of reducing the risk of developing ovarian cancer. A woman with a history of taking birth control pills for as little as one year has reduced her lifetime risk of developing ovarian cancer by at least 50%.

Anger sometimes is directed inwardly as the patient looks to blame herself for some perceived action such as eating processed foods or red meat. Sometimes anger is directed outwardly to her doctor who she believes should or should not have done something while under his/her care. Yet, realistically, the anger is misdirected as personal habits and extent of medical care have little impact on ovarian cancer risk in women, although they can affect risk of other pelvic malignancies. Cervical cancers, for example, are caused by Human Papillomavirus (HPV) infections resulting from sexual relations with an infected partner. They are largely prevented by the HPV vaccine and by having regular Pap smears. In the unvaccinated population, increased numbers of sexual partners are associated with an increased risk of cervical cancer. Uterine cancers are caused mainly by hormonal issues including excessive production of hormones caused by obesity or by taking unopposed estrogens for menopausal symptoms. This is one cancer for which diet or lifestyle can affect the risk. A diet which results in obesity or a sedentary lifestyle which also contributes to obesity results in an increased risk of uterine cancer. While discussing risks, I should mention that ovarian cancers are sometimes hereditary as in the BRCA families discussed previously, but are not the result of environmental factors or personal choices a woman makes. Likewise, uterine cancers can be related to genetic abnormalities, some of which are also associated with colon cancers (Lynch Syndrome). So, while anger is understandable, its target is elusive.

Anger towards the treating physician can arise if a cancer proves to be incurable. I recall an elderly woman sent to me with an early-stage cancer of the vulva. I performed the proper operation and based on well-established criteria expected her to be cured. There was no indication for any treatment beyond her surgery. Within a year her cancer recurred and in a matter of months following the recurrence, she died. Her daughter was furious because she felt something more should have been done after the operation. I explained to her that treatment criteria suggested a high probability of cure with the surgery I performed and that there was no additional advantage of follow up therapy in her mother's case. She would have none of it. She wrote a nasty report on the internet accusing me of being responsible for her mother's death. I felt terrible, mainly because my patient had died, but there was no assuaging her daughter's anger.

I think anger towards a physician just goes with the territory. Treatment outcomes are not always predictable and when the outcome is poor, the patient or her loved ones can lash out with their anger. If a physician is not prepared for anger directed towards him or her as he/she provides the best care possible, he/she probably should be in another line of work. Carnival workers, musicians, cruise directors and guides at theme parks rarely have anger directed towards them. Maybe that's where such an individual should look for employment rather than becoming a physician who cares for cancer patients.

BARGAINING. I really can't comment on "bargaining" except to note that, in women with terminal disease, bargaining to live a little longer to accomplish specific goals during end-of-life management can be very important. Physicians must be honest with their patients as they approach their final days, so they may set realistic short-term goals. Maybe it is important to live to see the birth of a grandchild, attend a graduation, or attend the wedding of a friend or relative. To the extent possible, efforts must be made to prolong life, even when the quality of life is poor, when such goals are attainable in the short term. Unrealistic goals must be identified as such. It might not be realistic to keep a patient with a bowel blockage alive for six weeks until the wedding of her favorite niece. Physicians often can prolong life of dying patients for days or weeks or even months at times through means such as intravenous nutritional support, aggressive management of failing kidneys or by performing a variety of surgical procedures. Such efforts must have a strong justification for patients with a terminal illness since the quality of life as the end-of-life approaches for these patients can be poor.

Justification for prolongation of the life of a terminally ill woman with severe pain, or having difficulty breathing, or with a bowel blockage can only be decided by the patient. I have had many patients who wanted to live until a family member could reach their bedside to say their goodbyes. I encourage them to do so hastily. I also suggest that they have their financial affairs in order and that their will and/or living trust be up to date. Such practical issues should be addressed while patients still have the capabilities to do so. Unfortunately, the bargain for living a little longer for these patients can be likened to a pact with the Devil. The value of living those additional days or weeks is typically offset by the terrible quality of life that many patients experience, and their families witness, in those final days.

DEPRESSION. Depression accompanies many women who are dealing with the stress of a cancer diagnosis and the treatments that the cancer necessitates. The removal of parts of a woman's body that are associated with gender identity is understandably depressing for so many women. Furthermore, side effects of chemotherapy including the loss of hair on the scalp and eyebrows, nausea, vomiting, and the constipation associated with many drugs can easily create a profound depression. I must say, however, that over the years, I have marveled at the strength of women who continue their roles as breadwinners, homemakers, caregivers, wives, mothers, and lovers as they fight their battles with cancer and its treatments. The world around them might be crumbling, but they are determined to be the foundation that keeps that world intact. That strength of character of women with gynecologic cancers is one aspect of the specialty that attracted me in the first place. Surprisingly few of my patients have found the need to take antidepressants although mild sedatives are sometimes helpful at night for these women. I do not recall a single patient who required hospitalization for depression over the many years of my career; however, many have requested referral for counseling which I have always encouraged and supported. These women manage to live their lives in the face of an uncertain outcome with dignity and purpose. It is easy to understand why I have been committed to my patients who live and die with dignity.

ACCEPTANCE: What do I mean by acceptance in the context of cancer care and the patients who must deal with this diagnosis and the uncertainty of their outcome? First there is the acceptance of the diagnosis, which of course is the opposite of denial. The overwhelming majority of newly diagnosed cancer patients I have cared for accept their diagnosis unquestionably. Their main objective is to understand what they can about the diagnosis and, more importantly, to have a plan of treatment as soon as possible. That goal is a healthy one and leads to the development of an important partnership between patient and physician. Initially, the physician serves as a source of valuable information and simultaneously becomes the Managing Partner of the partnership. There is one caveat, however. The patient is also a partner. The patient has the power of the veto. Accordingly, the Managing Partner must be persuasive for the partnership to move forward and offer the best treatment for the patient. Persuasion in this setting requires knowledge combined with sensitive and thoughtful discussion of the disease and its treatment options. Acceptance of the cancer diagnosis by the patient is implicit in this partnership.

The patient should exercise her responsibility to be proactive in her treatment by learning about her cancer and its treatment options. She should be prepared to tell her doctor "I need more information before I decide to move forward with my treatment" if that information has not been forthcoming. I expand on that discussion in Chapter 27 entitled Control and Uncertainty.

As treatment evolves and the extent of the cancer is determined, a new type of acceptance might be required. All the parties in this partnership dedicated to treating a woman with cancer are doing their best for a favorable outcome. However, information at the initial evaluation of the cancer or new information that arises with the passage of time during or after initial treatment might indicate that a favorable outcome is not likely. Then another type of acceptance is necessary, acceptance of cancer progression and probable resultant death. Acceptance in this setting is not the same as surrender and waiting for death. Rather it is a positive step that allows recognition of the circumstances and permits one to see things as they are rather than where the patient would like them to be. By this understanding it is possible to move forward and accomplish activities that are important to the patient over the time she still has. Perhaps she will want to visit a place she has always dreamed of seeing, or get together with old friends she has not seen for years, or reconcile differences with family members over long standing disagreements. In my opinion, it is unconscionable, to withhold unfavorable prognostic information from a patient in the belief that she will not be able to process the information and move forward. The responsibility of the physician at these times is to be able to provide unfavorable information in a supportive and hopeful manner while not providing inaccurate information creating false hopes. I have addressed this issue in greater detail in the final chapter.

Failure of a patient to embrace acceptance when she is incurable is overwhelming to the psyche and adversely affects one's quality of life. It requires too much negative energy to deny acceptance, and denial prevents one from experiencing joy. Focusing on the negative does not allow one to experience the joyfulness of a sunset, or a baby's first steps, or the sound of rain on a roof, or snow on the needles of a pine tree after a winter snowstorm. By accepting the reality of the condition, each moment is more precious and provides an opportunity for happiness. This is the time for one to practice gratitude for all the good that has happened during one's life and to wash away the negatives. This is an opportunity to practice kindness with loved ones even people one does not know. Because kindness itself is joyful. This is a time to spend with family doing ordinary things that people who care for each other do together. This is a time for picnics or visiting a zoo or playing croquet or learning needlepoint. There is no reason that an incurable patient with cancer cannot enjoy her life even when it is shorter than she wishes it to be.

Let me tell you about Joan. She will always be one of my favorite patients, but I must confess that she is in a large club in that regard, because I have had lots of favorite patients over the many years of my practice. Joan had an advanced cancer that had started in her ovaries. This was another unusual one, a granulosa cell tumor. These cancers tend to be early stage and easily curable in most instances; however, hers was different in that it had already spread when it was diagnosed. I didn't take care of her early on during her cancer treatment. In fact, she was first diagnosed many years before I first met her. Characteristic of these cancers is a long life for patients even when incurable. In fact, some women have gone 25 or 30 years with a granulosa cell tumor before it recurred.

I first met Joan around 2012 when she came to see me in consultation. She let me know right off that she was used to overseeing her care and that she knew a lot about her disease as well as her treatment options. She knew she had cancer in the abdomen, that she was not curable, and she told me so. She wanted a doctor who would work with her and respect her wishes, within reason, and give her a good quality of life for as long as she had to live. I told her I could work with that, and then she told me she liked me because I was honest with her and showed her respect.

I recall that initial consultation as if it were just a few days ago. Joan was accepting of her condition and wanted a partnership that would maximize her time and her quality of life. I thought she was an ideal patient since I love it when patients take such an active role in the management of their disease. Joan told me that she was a member of a group of women with this rare type of cancer and that they served as a support group as well as a source of up-to-date information about treatment advancements. I told her I would be glad to review any materials she provided me from the group but that I would need to make recommendations based on my best clinical judgement rather than some new and untried treatment that might come along. She told me that she was fine with that as well.

I took care of Joan from that initial encounter in 2012 until her death on December 15, 2017. Initially I did a massive tumor resection on her that removed much but not all of her cancer. During the five years I cared for her I saw her every couple of months. She was usually accompanied by her husband. During that time, we did a variety of chemotherapy treatments after her surgery when her cancer recurred in the abdomen and in the chest cavity (space around the lungs). Some of the various treatments helped briefly. Some did not seem to provide much, if any, benefit.

As her cancer progressed, she developed an increasing shortness of breath. She requested that fluid be removed from her abdomen, which I arranged. She also requested removal of fluid from her chest for comfort, which I also arranged. She did have progressive pain but was adamantly opposed to narcotics for pain relief. This was the only area where I had a disagreement with her as I wanted to provide greater comfort measures for her. She viewed narcotics as the beginning of the end for her and she did not want to face that yet. She won out as she usually did. Remember, patients have the veto. Up until the end, she remained in control, focused on her personal goals which revolved around her close-knit family.

Joan never asked "why me" or expressed anger or complained to me. She was always respectful and thankful for the care she received. I was saddened when her husband sent me a note that Joan had died December 15, 2017. He asked if I would come to a memorial service a month after her passing. I really do not like funerals or memorial services, possibly because it is a reminder of my own mortality. In my line of work, I really didn't need more reminders of just how short our time here will be. Accordingly, I do not usually go to funerals or memorial services. However, I made an exception for this special woman. It was important to her family that I attend, and I had established a strong bond with her husband, so I did attend the memorial service to which I was invited. Joan was in her mid-50s when she died, on her own terms.

I will share two notes she sent me during the final months of her life because I think they illustrate the kind of person she was and the relationship that we shared as doctor and patient. The first one is dated May 2015, two and a half years before she died. She sent this to me shortly after an office visit at which time she was doing less well than over the previous months and was experiencing increasing abdominal pain. She had lost her composure briefly and wanted to share her feelings with me about that office visit.

> Dear Dr. Berman,
>
> I want to apologize for breaking down in your office tonight. I just don't want to be at the end of my road with my disease. I feel like pain management is the beginning of the end for me, and I am not yet ready to face that. I have always tried to remain poised, and in control in your office. I realize what a difficult job you have at times and I never want to make it

any more difficult for you. It must be hard to watch women suffer knowing that some...many, will not survive their disease. You are a skilled surgeon that came highly recommended, and a man with a huge heart. You may not remember our beginning, but you were a 2nd opinion for me, that I ended up preferring to my treating physician. I will never forget your willingness to dig in and try to go for the best possible resection of my disease. Even though it didn't go as we all had hoped, it still gave me great relief once I healed from the extensive surgery for a couple of years. It was still worth every effort as far as I am concerned.

Thank you for the kindness you have always shown me. I appreciate you more than you can know.

Sincerely, Joan

The second email note was March 25, 2017, which was nine months before she died. She was in hospice and feeling better, mainly because of improved pain management. She had delayed taking narcotics for a few years until she finally went into hospice.

Hi Dr. Berman,

I wanted to check in with you and say hello. Being on hospice has been a very good experience for me. In the beginning, the pain relief was so amazing, I rallied and felt great, almost too good. While I was under your care, I fought taking anything narcotic honestly for a few reasons, mostly because I was the caretaker of both of my parents, and I do not believe in driving under the influence of anything. I suffered too long, and wish circumstances had been different. My parents made my life extremely difficult, but I honored my mom, was with her when she took her last breath, and then, it was time for me to focus on my own suffering.

It has not been easy, my demented father lives beneath on the first floor, and after mom passed, I was very much thrown into caring almost full time for him. Thankfully, my oldest daughter has really stepped up and we have found live-in care for him. What a relief.

I have had a few really bad spells (for lack of a better word), and of course my journey is slowly coming to an end, but I am still trying to find ways to enjoy my life, and my friends and family have been very loving and supportive.

I really wanted to let you know, I am still alive and I am trying not to give anyone too much grief :) Thank you for all that you have done for me. I appreciate you and think very highly of you. Not only are you a great doctor and skilled surgeon, you have a huge heart, which I felt in the beginning when I first became your patient. As I learned about all of the wonderful things you do, helping so many people, working to help people who otherwise would have no care, I was moved very deeply when you shared with me what a typical week involved for you. You sure do move around, and you help so many people.

I think it must be a very difficult job dealing with people who are terminally ill. It must be hard to stay detached enough to be able to help people and not lose your mind when so many of us fail to respond to treatment.

One thing that I especially appreciated about you is that you were willing to listen to me, and you took me seriously, would actually read the abstracts that I brought in and actually prescribed medicines for me. With your good judgement, and with research, you were willing to do so much to help me. It is nearly impossible to find a doctor that is even remotely willing to do anything like that. Thank you for giving me the time of day, and showing me kindness and respect. Thank you for having a heart bigger than your whole self and for leading with kindness and love, and not from an egotistical place. You are a kind and gentle man who showed me great compassion and respect.

Thank you for all of those things, and for all that you continue to do to help others. I appreciate you more than you can ever imagine.

Wishing you much happiness and thinking of you with a heart full of gratitude.

Sincerely, Joan

Even as I write this book, I am moved to tears re-reading Joan's correspondence. She was such a thoughtful woman. It is easy to see why she has been one of my favorite patients. She lived life to the fullest and accepted her disease with dignity and without regret or compromise. Joan's acceptance of her disease and its unfavorable prognosis was critical to permitting her to enjoy her remaining days.

CHAPTER FOURTEEN

HUMILITY
LAURA, JANIS AND ROSEMARY

Humility is such an important and worthy attribute. That is why I want to address it. A book such as this one would be incomplete without addressing humility. Humility is the belief that one is not better than others. It is also the acknowledgement of the worth of others. It requires an ability to understand one's strengths and weaknesses as an individual. People admire others for their humility, for being modest in action and speech, and for being unpretentious in their behavior. We often reject those who are boastful, especially when that boastfulness is designed to impress others about their own self-worth. Humility demonstrates a wish to become better. That should be a goal all of us set because all of us can improve upon ourselves in many ways.

By being humble we acknowledge our shortcomings and suggest that we are trying to overcome them rather than accept them. Remarkably, humility does not exclude self-confidence. In contrast, there is a broad divide between self-confidence and boastfulness. Humility and self-confidence are felt inwardly. Boastfulness is expressed outwardly. Self-confidence is a positive thought process while boastfulness is a negative action. People who are humble typically are grateful for what they have and for what they have accomplished. Those who are boastful are merely trying to convince others that they know a great deal, have financial worth, or have accomplished great things. They typically are not grateful for what they have accumulated or have accomplished. They typically have an inflated ego and sense of self-importance. Knowledgeable and accomplished individuals usually are not boastful. Humble individuals tend to have better relationships with their peers and loved ones than those who are not. They tend to put others first, are more caring and empathetic, more commonly are good listeners, tend not to be the center of attention, are respectful of others, and usually exhibit a high degree of curiosity. Humility fosters gratitude. These are all desirable goals that we should aspire to.

Caring for women with cancers is a humbling career choice. We lose the battle as often as we win. Sometimes we lose when we expect to win and sometimes, we win when we expect to lose. Clearly, we are not in total control of the outcome of our patients. If effort assured success, all our patients would do well; however, that simply is not the way it works. That observation alone is humbling.

While I have always had a great deal of self-confidence, I believe that I exhibit humility and am not boastful. Still, I am not so sure that I have always exhibited humility; however, the past 50 years of my professional life have certainly conspired to make me so. I do not assume that I am the smartest or the best at what I do but I know that I always do my best for my patients without regard to financial gain or other possible benefit to me. I have never objected to a patient seeking out another opinion after I have given mine and gladly care for patients who have questioned my wisdom and sought others for advice before choosing to return to me for care. I have never told a patient I am the best doctor for women with gynecologic cancers or that I have special skills unique to me. When a patient tells me she has chosen me because she was told or read that I was the best doctor for her type of cancer, I typically suggest that there are many fine physicians who could care for her but that I am glad that she has chosen me to be her doctor. I always tried to manage my patients in a fashion that is knowledgeable, caring, compassionate, empathetic, honest, and humble. I always tried to make time to sit and talk with my patients about their fears and wishes.

Let me tell you about two patients whose devotion and trust in me as their doctor has been humbling. I guess my story that I shared of Joan's journey would have qualified in this regard; however, I would like to share the stories of two other remarkable women. First, let me tell you about Laura who is married to Len. Len is a medical equipment sales professional. He supplies radiological equipment and devices used by radiation therapists. Laura and Len are originally from Cleveland, Ohio where they visit for several months each year to be with family. They have five adult children and, at last count, thirteen grandchildren.

When Laura was diagnosed with an aggressive type of uterine cancer at 58 years of age in 2007, Len asked all his professional contacts in medicine who should see Laura. Ultimately, they came to see me. Cancers of the uterus are evaluated as to their aggressiveness which is called the grade of the cancer. There are three grades and hers was the worst, grade-three. Whereas most uterine cancers are grade 1 and highly curable because they typically do not spread to other areas of the body, grade-three tumors can spread early and recur often, so the prognosis is uncertain.

When I evaluated Laura, the best evidence based on her exam and radiologic studies was that her cancer had not spread internally. I recommended surgery for her treatment and also to help determine if there was occult spread not detected on her preoperative assessment. I performed a complete hysterectomy removing her uterus, ovaries, and tubes. I also removed all the lymph nodes in the pelvis and some outside the pelvis. The cancer appeared very aggressive microscopically but there was no evidence of spread in any of the tissues I had removed. I was delighted for her and was planning additional therapy because of her high risk of the cancer recurring. Such recurrences happen, typically several months up to a couple of years following surgery.

Laura returned to see me for her six-week checkup. I was astounded to find that her cancer had already recurred, even before I was able to initiate further therapy. There was a tumor mass in the vagina which had not been present six weeks earlier; an obvious recurrence. I evaluated her further with a biopsy to confirm the recurrence and ordered appropriate scans which did not provide evidence of cancer elsewhere. I recommended radiation therapy to her pelvis to attack the area of recurrence and planned on chemotherapy after completion of the radiation because of a high risk of recurrences elsewhere in her body. Chemotherapy drugs pass into all organs and all cells within the organs of the patient undergoing treatment. If cancer cells were elsewhere but not seen on imaging, my hope was that the chemotherapy would destroy those cells and effect a cure. Her husband, Len, went to his sources in southern California who suggested radiation treatments in San Diego which was not too far from where they lived. This was accomplished over six weeks followed by internal radiation focused primarily on the vaginal tumor as well. She came back to see me. The mass was gone after radiation. I started her on a course of intensive chemotherapy which she tolerated remarkably well except for the expected hair loss, nausea, vomiting, constipation, etc. that I discussed elsewhere.

I began seeing Laura after completion of her chemotherapy at three-month intervals checking for possible signs of recurrence of the cancer, and less frequently after two years of negative follow up examinations. Laura has remained cancer free since then for the past 13 years. She continues to keep me updated around Christmastime each year. As I look back, it is hard for me to believe that her cancer recurred so quickly after her operation and then, equally surprising, that she has been cured. Both the early recurrence and the resulting cure after radiation and chemotherapy were unlikely, yet the ultimate outcome was what we had hoped for. We definitely had walked down the good luck side of the street.

There are a couple of other interesting observations of Laura and Len that I can share. They have been back to Cleveland almost every year since I began taking care of her. When there, she also goes to the Cleveland Clinic for any needed testing. She could have chosen to be treated there, but she had done her research and was confident that I would give her the best possible care. The other interesting note is that while Laura was doing fabulously well, her husband, the picture of health when I first met Laura, developed a cancer of the kidney that spread to his brain. Remarkably, he has done well for at least four years, but remains under treatment with one of the newer biological drugs developed to treat many types of cancer.

I like to share correspondence from my patients when appropriate, so I have a few notes from Laura, two of which I will copy here. One was written about a year after I first began caring for her, around 2008, and the second was in 2014, just a few months after my wife, Marlene, died. I often share my own story with many of my patients, and Joan and Len knew that Marlene had been ill and had died after a lengthy and disabling illness. I believe that sharing my own story with my patients brings me closer to them and confirms that I am just another human with children, grandchildren, a wife, friends, happiness and sadness, just as they are. I enjoy sitting and chatting with my patients and getting to know them on a personal level. In so many ways, I am just like my patients.

Her first note:

> Dr. Berman,
>
> My husband, Len and I interviewed and researched to find the best surgeon and oncologist and thank God we found you! We are so grateful for your skill and knowledge and your caring concern. May this holiday (Christmas) be especially filled with joy and love for you and your wife as it is for us. You will be in our prayers.
>
> With much fondness, Laura

Her second note after Marlene's passing:

> Dr. Berman, Len and I have thought of you so often always, but especially since the passing of your wife. How blessed she was to have such a devoted and caring husband. Your grief and loneliness must be profound. Thank God you have such a loving family and successful practice...please don't leave us for a while...I know everyone loves you!
>
> With much prayer and fondness, Laura and Len

My second story regarding humility is of Janis who is married to Nathan. Her sister is Rosemary. Janis is a registered nurse who works in the office of a busy Obstetrician Gynecologist in Orange County, California. She was in her early 40s with a young son and daughter when I first met her in 1999 as a new patient. She presented with a large pelvic mass. Findings suggested an advanced ovarian cancer. I counseled Janis and Nathan about the likely diagnosis and the need for surgery. We scheduled surgery within a week or two. My suspicion was correct that this was an advanced ovarian cancer. I found spread to multiple areas of the abdomen and pelvis including the ovaries, tubes, uterus, surface of the large and small intestine, omentum and multiple other areas as well. I was able to remove all the cancer except an area lying directly over the pancreas. I didn't feel I could remove that area safely. She tolerated the surgery well and recovered in a few days.

I began Janis on a course of chemotherapy within three weeks of her operation and after six courses of treatment recommended that I take her back to surgery to see if there was still residual cancer present. I had arranged for a surgical oncologist to be present so the region that had contained cancer at the end of the first operation could be removed, if necessary. In those days, more than 20 years ago, "second look" operations similar to that which I was recommending were done frequently in such circumstances. Now we know that such second operations do not improve the likelihood of cure, so they are rarely done any longer. Happily, there was no evidence of residual cancer at Janis' second operation and no further therapy was indicated. Still, most such patients, even with no cancer found at the second operation, have a cancer recurrence at a later date, but Janis was lucky. She has remained cancer free for more than two decades. Understandably, she and Nathan are most grateful to me.

A year after Janis underwent her operation and completion of chemotherapy, her sister, Rosemary, came to see me with Janis at my UCI office. She was afraid that she was at high risk for ovarian cancer because of her sister's diagnosis at a young age. Most women with ovarian cancers are postmenopausal at diagnosis and those who are premenopausal are somewhat more likely to have a BRCA gene that was responsible for the development of the cancer. I tried to reassure her that her risk was low as her sister's BRCA test was negative, but she had decided she wanted a hysterectomy and that she would have another surgeon do it if I was unwilling. The indication for her operation was marginal at best, but I told her I would submit the request to her insurance company, expecting that they would deny the prophylactic surgery. Surprisingly, her insurance carrier thought that it was reasonable and authorized the surgery, which I performed on Rosemary in the summer of 2001. She lived in New York but had flown out to have me do her operation. She did well as expected as she did not have cancer and, to my knowledge, is still doing well, back in New York.

Both of my patients, Laura and Janis (plus Rosemary) have honored me by their gratitude, their respect, their loyalty and their kindness. If that does not create joy and humility for a physician, I do not know what would. As with Laura, I will share notes I received from Janis and Rosemary.

From Janis one year after her operations:

> Dear Dr. Berman,
>
> I have begun this thank you note so many times and often give up part way as I have found it so difficult to express in words my total gratefulness for all you have done for me over this last year.
>
> I want to thank you first of all for my life. I hoped and prayed that I would survive ovarian cancer and although I know we're not in remission, it feels so incredible to be where I am today. I am so grateful for your skill as a surgeon and for your commitment to medicine and research that has helped get me here. As an RN I had worked with MDs from UCI and I had always thought they were the best. Now as a patient I now know you all are the BEST! I cannot believe how incredible the care I have received has been.
>
> Thank you most of all for your care for me and for all the time you have taken to help educate me, my husband (and now my sister too!) toward the process of healing. You could not have been more wonderful to us and we have valued your kindness and gentleness to us both. We value and respect your wisdom and are thankful we get to continue in your care. With very grateful hearts.
>
> Always, Janis and Nathan

Then the next note was written on the back of a preprinted card which read "Please celebrate, along with us, our FIVE-year Anniversary mark. Thank You for everything"

The note begins:

> Dear Dr. Berman, I am so grateful for your commitment to my care that you have shown over the last FIVE years. I have felt so blessed to be under your care and to have a physician so deeply committed to the advancement of medical treatments. I am grateful for topotecan!! (one of the chemotherapy drugs she had received on a clinical trial sponsored by the Gynecologic Oncology Group for women with advanced ovarian cancers). It was my prayer to make it to the five-year mark-to see my son married and my daughter graduated from high school and headed off to college. I guess I should have asked for MORE! Thank you for always being caring and positive in a field of medicine that must have its days. Our hearts are deeply knit with yours.
>
> Thank you. Janis and Nathan

And then the third note dated March 6, 2007, now eight years after her treatment:

> Dear Dr. Berman, I don't know if you have other patients that come in contact with as many people with ovarian cancer as I do but I feel as though I see an abundance. The only good thing about it is I know an incredible physician and surgeon-you!
>
> Working in Dr. X's office gives me additional opportunity to "brag" about you. Hearing you share with the Jones' post surgically was amazing. (This was a friend with ovarian cancer that Janis referred to me) You share so clearly and with such compassion. Of course, I wasn't there when you shared with my family, but Nathan tells me you were very kind and tender. What a very tough job you have. I appreciate your work in my life almost daily. Thank you. I was in awe today so grateful for physicians like you who care and practice incredible medicine. Thank you sounds so minimal, but I just couldn't let tonight pass without telling you once again-thank you.
>
> Janis, R.N. (and cancer survivor!)

And finally, the note from Rosemary after her hysterectomy August 8, 2001:

> Dear Dr. Berman, Thank you for being such a caring, tender doctor. I know that my case was tiny compared to my sister's, but you treated me with such respect. I am amazed at how well I feel! I am only two days post-op and today I took a quick ride to Costco with Janis, and even watered the garden! I had no pain, only very bearable discomfort (I've had worse menstrual pain!)
>
> I have admired you for a year, since you helped Janis so much. But now I have my own reason to say...Thank you.
>
> A loyal patient, Rosemary

Janis, Nathan, and Rosemary are special people. Their confidence in me, their gratitude, kindness and love are all I have hoped to receive from my patients. Even more remarkable to me is the outpouring of thanks I have received over the years from surviving spouses and children of patients who were less fortunate and died of their disease despite my efforts in caring for them. Knowing that they appreciated my efforts for their loved ones, even when unsuccessful, helped to lessen the loss I felt when a patient died.

I can't begin to express all the feelings a physician experiences when a patient dies. There is an intense sadness. There is a feeling of failure. There is a profound sense of loss. There is a feeling of empathy for the family of the deceased. And there is so much more. It is not surprising to understand that depression and physician burnout with early retirement is so common among those of us who care for oncology patients. Even physician suicide is disproportionately high among oncologists. Developing coping tools is critical to the mental wellbeing of physicians just as it is for our patients. Yet medical schools, residency programs and fellowship programs have been notoriously lacking in discussing the issue and in providing helpful tools to prevent physician burnout. It's just an unfortunate shortcoming of physician training at every phase of the process of education.

CHAPTER FIFTEEN

HUMOR
The Bag Lady and Jun

As in all aspects of life, humor is important, even when the subject is a serious one. The ability to laugh even when the going gets rough is an important coping mechanism that helps us deal with life's challenges. And the ability to laugh at oneself is an important measure of health and well-being. When I laugh at myself, I am reminded of my flaws and allows me to make light of them. That is a positive response to my shortcomings. And all of us have shortcomings. I still remember going out to a party with friends around age 20, too young to be drinking alcohol, but enjoying a screwdriver (vodka and orange juice). It tasted so good and I really liked orange juice and the vodka made me feel as if I was the life of the party. So, I had a second and a third and maybe even a fourth one. The next day I was so sick I had to spend most of the morning with knees flexed, my chest over the toilet bowl as my GI tract kept reminding me that I was an idiot. To this day I have never again mixed vodka with orange juice and rarely drink orange juice, but I do like good vodka. It is so easy to transport myself back to that party and laugh at myself trying to show my alcohol tolerance to my friends while becoming the life of the party, in my mind only.

I have enjoyed so much humor in my practice over the years. I have loved laughing with my patients and sometimes laughing at circumstances that patient care has provided. I continue to love reading some of the notes sent to me that make me laugh. I have kept most of the notes sent to me by patients over the years. I thought I might share a couple to illustrate my point.

The first brief note requires an introduction. In operating on women with advanced cancers, at times I have had to remove a portion of the rectum in order to give the best chance for a cure. This is especially true for ovarian cancers. Usually, I can reconnect the rectum to the lower colon in such circumstances, but at times that cannot be done safely at the time of surgery. Such patients must live with a colostomy and eliminate stool into a bag worn on the exterior abdominal wall. While this can be permanent, whenever possible, I try to reverse the colostomy at a second operation to eliminate the bag. That second operation typically is done after several months and usually following completion of chemotherapy. When colostomy reversal can be done successfully, the patient is incredibly grateful, as you might expect. With that background, I received a brief note from just such a patient whose colostomy I had closed several weeks earlier.

The note read:

> It's one of life's perks when your bottom works!
>
> With thanks from an ex-bag-lady.
>
> Mary

I also received a hilarious note from one of my patients I cared for in Pittsburgh around 1978. For about 13 or 14 years she carried around guilt because she had not been totally honest with me when I was taking care of her. She was concerned that her dishonesty had harmed me in some way, so finally in 1992, 14 years later, she got it off her chest. She sent me a note. As you might guess from the content she was not from the United States and English was not her first language. She was from Taiwan where I've heard being dishonest with your doctor is a definite no-no.

The letter reads as follows:

> Dear Dr. Michael Berman,
>
> My name is Jun. I was a patient of yours at the Meeky Women's Hospital (sic, Magee Women's Hospital) in Pittsburgh. You removed a tumor in my uterus. My husband and I are very thankful for what you did for me.
>
> Last year during a checkup, my doctor told me you were still teaching. I commented that you were a very good, responsible doctor and he seemed surprised that you were not leading a better life. Secondly my son decided not to become a doctor because there is too much responsibility. These two factors made me write this letter.
>
> I am writing to let you know how sorry I am that I didn't tell you before the surgery that in Taiwan I had previously had plastic surgery on my vagina before came U.S.A. After the surgery, you had also asked me several times if I had hurt my back. I always told you that I had not, even though when I was three I had in fact damaged it. I decided to write this letter after so many years, because I have always been sorry that I didn't tell you the truth, and I am worried that you suffered as a result. I am very sorry, and I hope you can forgive me. May God bless you.
>
> Sincerely,
>
> Jun

Now I should mention that this patient for years sent me gifts after I moved from Pittsburgh, Pennsylvania to Southern California. I don't know how she got my address; however, she was resourceful and sent me something about once a year. I think she stopped sending them to me after she got this off her chest and no longer felt guilty about her dishonesty The gifts had been sent to me as a kind of peace offering after not being completely honest with me when I first met her. I often pull that letter out of my desk drawer when I really want a laugh.

CHAPTER SIXTEEN

RESPONSIBILITY
JANE, DONNA, KERRY AND SAPPHIRE

Choosing to become a physician assumes a willingness to accept great responsibility for the care of others. Physicians pledge to be responsible to make correct diagnoses, to administer proper treatment, to choose what is right for the patient without consideration for what is best for oneself, to remain updated about advancements in medicine, to respect the privacy of our patients, and to deal with them equitably and honestly. All these responsibilities are stated or implied in the Hippocratic Oath of physician ethical standards which can be summarized by the pledge *primin non nocere* or "first do no harm." This pledge not to do harm in the broader sense should be adopted as a personal commitment from all of us, not just physicians. It is a way of restating the "golden rule" of treating others as we wish to be treated. All of us should choose the responsible way of living our lives. There is a famous story of two rabbis, Hillel and Shammai, who were challenged to teach the Jewish Bible (the Tanakh) while standing on one foot. Their response was to recite the golden rule. We should choose our friends carefully, selecting those who also practice responsibility as a way of life. We should commit to being honest and loyal, being humble and forgiving, being creative, compassionate and hard working. These are responsibilities all of us should aspire to.

As a physician treating young women and even adolescents with cancers at times, my sense of personal responsibility was especially great. These patients often had not yet had the chance to have children. They hoped I would be able to treat their cancers successfully while preserving their fertility. Sometimes that was not possible. You might recall the young woman in denial who had cervical cancer and refused therapy because her fertility could not be saved. She chose to die from a treatable cancer rather than give up something so precious to her. But sometimes it is possible to treat a young woman with a gynecologic cancer and still preserve fertility. This is especially true for women with an unusual type of ovarian cancer—a germ cell tumor.

Actually, there are several types of germ cell tumors; however, almost all of them can be treated conservatively with removal of the affected ovary while saving the opposite ovary and preserving fertility in most instances. I should mention that these tumors historically have been lethal with poor survival rates until effective chemotherapy was developed that proved to be curative. For example, one type of germ cell tumor called a yolk sac tumor or endodermal sinus tumor, was associated with a 15% cure rate for the earliest stage prior to chemotherapy. These tumors now are virtually 100% curable with modern chemotherapy for early-stage disease (cancer confined to one ovary); even with widespread disease, the majority of such women are curable. This remarkable observation is a result of clinical trials of women with these types of cancers who were treated largely in Cancer Centers throughout the United States. In fact, most of the advancements in cancer therapeutics has resulted from such clinical trials in which patients with incurable cancers are treated with novel therapies that over a course of many years prove to be more effective than standard therapies currently in existence.

Over the years some of the nicest follow up notes I have received have come from young women with ovarian germ cell cancers that I treated while they were still adolescents or young adults. Those notes often have been accompanied by a photograph of themselves with their husbands and even with children of their own. A handwritten Post-It from my former patient, Jane, diagnosed with a germ cell cancer as a young teenager, accompanied a beautiful photograph of her with her two young sons, handsome and blue eyed just like Jane and her husband.

It read:

> I want you to have this (photograph) because without you and the decisions you helped my parents with, this would not have been possible. You are in my thoughts always!
>
> Thank you! Love, Jane

Another beautiful note was sent by Donna on March 1, 1997, 13 years after I took care of her with a malignant germ cell tumor of the ovary. She was living in Phoenix, Arizona and sent it with two photographs: one of her wedding in Long Beach in 1992 and the other of her two-year-old son who was born in 1995. In her note she reminded me that she was my patient in 1984 at which time she was nineteen and diagnosed with ovarian cancer.

She told me,

> "I have been wanting to write and tell you how I've been doing but never seemed to have the time." She was "happy to say that I've been fine ever since my last surgery back in Feb 1984. I married in June 1992 to an Englishman and lived in London for two years until I found out that I was pregnant (surprise to me)." She also said "I'm happy to say that we had a nine-pound baby boy born on January 26, 1995 at St Joseph hospital. Not bad for a lady who had just turned thirty in November 1994...At present I'm living in Phoenix where my husband works as an accountant and I'm enjoying the pleasure of raising our son..."
>
> Sincerely, Donna

Every physician's goal is to snatch a patient out of harm's way, to cure a terrible cancer, to win against the odds. But here are two very young ladies with cancers who have been able to move on and live normal productive, happy lives. They have married and have had families of their own. They have lived to love and be loved. Such a blessing!

One final note I would like to share came from Kerry, which was not her birth name. She had been born Frances. Her relationship with her mother was apparently explosive around the time of her cancer diagnosis and treatment when Kerry was 13 years old. At some point after surgery and chemotherapy, Kerry decided to live with her now-divorced father who was very supportive and loving. She changed her name to Kerry because she wanted to separate her new life with her father from her prior life with her mother. Living with her mother sounded pretty toxic. As with Donna and Jane, Kerry had a similarly aggressive germ cell tumor that I operated on and then treated with chemotherapy in the 1990's. As with Donna and Jane, I removed the affected ovary but did not remove her uterus or her other ovary. She had done well physically but had lots of emotional issues, some related to her cancer and some to her home situation.

I had not seen Kerry for several years after which she sent me a note letting me know that she was doing well and was moving on in her life. She was now living in Idaho with her father. She sent me a Christmas note many years ago, probably prior to 2000, in which she wrote:

> Christmas greetings to you and yours. Things up here in Idaho are going well. I am so excited this will be the first white Christmas that I will remember. Thanks again for all of your help in the past. I will never forget you, nor my dad, and I know the Lord surely won't.
>
> God Bless you Dr. Berman,
>
> Love, Kerry

She added a P.S. that read:

> My health is doing better! I feel much better than the last time I saw you. Also, I now go by Kerry as opposed to Fran. Next time I see you I will elaborate.

Kerry had moved on beyond the cancer which, to her mind, was likely less threatening than her home situation had been. When I saw her again several years after her cancer treatment, she had gained a great deal of weight, likely a result of the stresses she had been dealing with. Her life was not perfect but improving. I was so happy to see that she was in a good place physically and, I believe, emotionally. I had been her doctor and now I was a caring observer as she was dealing with the ghosts of her past life. I have thought of Kerry many times over the years. I wish her only happiness. I have always tried to provide emotional support for my patients during and even long after I have actively cared for them. All my patients are unique and special, but the children and adolescents have a special place in my heart.

There is one other story of a young woman with ovarian cancer that I would also like to share. Her situation was different from Donna, Jane and Kerry. We will call her Sapphire. Sapphire was four months pregnant when she was sent to me with an obvious ovarian cancer based on her physical examination, ultrasound test and a markedly elevated CA-125 measurement. She had never been pregnant. She and her husband had been trying to have a child for a couple of years. Her excitement about her pregnancy was replaced by grief and heartache when she learned of her cancer diagnosis. I explained to her that she would require surgery to treat the cancer; however, it might be possible to preserve the pregnancy. Even though a pregnancy relies on the ovary from which ovulation had occurred to support the developing pregnancy in early months, by the fourth month removal of the ovaries typically would not likely cause an abortion. I anticipated removing both ovaries as well as the omentum and lymph nodes in the pelvis and abdomen as I suspected that the cancer was advanced. If there was cancer on the surface of the uterus, my plan was to remove the surface involvement, but not the uterus with its contained pregnancy and fetus. Sapphire agreed to this plan. Under no circumstance would I be able to remove the uterus based on our agreement preoperatively. Sapphire and her husband were counseled about the possibility of the surgery inducing an abortion; however, this was still a much safer approach than waiting another four months until such time that we could be confident that the pregnancy would provide a viable infant.

I performed the operation outlined. There was limited spread of the cancer which I was able to remove surgically. The pregnancy did not abort. Her recovery was uneventful. Unfortunately, because of the nature and extent of her cancer, she required chemotherapy to maximize her chance of cure. I didn't feel that we could wait safely until she delivered her baby and recommended that we begin a course of chemotherapy while she was still pregnant. I reassured her that the fetal organs were already developed and therefore the risk of fetal abnormalities from the chemotherapy was low. Understandably she was apprehensive about starting chemotherapy while still pregnant, but statistics show that the risks to the fetus from chemotherapy at this point in the pregnancy was minimal.

Fetal abnormalities from chemotherapy are common earlier in pregnancy, but not after the third month. Furthermore, the particular drugs that she would require are not those likely to cause fetal problems at any time during a pregnancy. Again, we reached an agreement to proceed. I began chemotherapy about the beginning of her fifth month of pregnancy. She received four of the planned six courses of treatment which brought her to about eight months.

At that time, I stopped the chemotherapy because of risks to Sapphire and possibly the infant if she delivered during the first three weeks following chemotherapy. I was concerned that the chemotherapy drug effect on the platelets of both the fetus and Sapphire might place her and the fetus at risk for hemorrhage with delivery, so we had to stop the treatment temporarily until after she delivered her infant. She delivered uneventfully after which I gave her the remaining two courses of chemotherapy. Her final treatment was completed in early 2011. Sapphire sent me a note at Christmas that year which read:

> Dr. Berman,
>
> Thank you for saving my life as well as my baby's life. We have so much to give thanks this year and we definitely will celebrate more birthdays and Christmases.
>
> Thanks to you! Merry X'mas and Happy New Year,
>
> Sincerely, Sapphire

Because I needed to remove both of Sapphire's ovaries during her cancer operation, she has been on hormone replacement therapy for more than a decade. She was still of premenopausal age, so I started her on birth control pills (oral contraceptive pill—OCP) for hormone replacement. She certainly did not need them for contraception, since she had no ovaries, but the OCP's served as an effective means of preventing hot flashes and osteoporosis. Sapphire keeps up with me at least yearly and has sent me pictures of her son on several occasions. He is a couple of inches shorter than expected for his age, and that could be an effect of the chemotherapy he had been exposed to while in utero. In any case he and his mom are well and thriving.

Sapphire, her husband, and son live in Florida. Her last contact in November 2020 was in a note sent to my nurse, Sandy. Sandy had helped coordinate Sapphire's surgery and then her chemotherapy.

She wrote:

> Hi Sandy, How are you? Pray that you had a Happy Thanksgiving. I have been thinking about you, Kathy (our surgery scheduler, medical assistant and friend of most of my patients) and Dr. Berman a lot and I am very thankful of your love and care while I was under Dr. Berman's treatment. Please send my sincere grateful regards to Dr. Berman and Kathy if they do not receive this email. When it's safe to travel; I'd love to stop by.
>
> Wish you all a wonderful Thanksgiving & Merry Christmas

She sent the note with a photograph of Sapphire and her son, who looks just like his mom.

Shakespeare's play, *All's Well that Ends Well*, sums up the story of Sapphire and her family. As Shakespeare might have said, the problems and pitfalls of an enterprise are justified and forgotten, so long as everything turns out well in the end. And it did.

CHAPTER SEVENTEEN

HONESTY : CHRISTINE

I have mentioned honesty a couple of times in the context of communication with patients, but I have not really focused on its importance in medicine, just as in life. Maybe I have taken for granted that whoever reads this book accepts and embraces the value of honesty and its importance, but maybe I should not be so naïve. Let me just state that honesty is one of the most important qualities that an individual should exhibit. It is the basis on which character is defined. The word "honor" is the root of honesty and, as such, lack of honesty suggests a lack of honor. Lack of honesty is a serious character flaw.

Perhaps I am too severe in my characterization. Does telling a white lie equate with dishonesty and a lack of honor? Certainly not, because lies designed to protect another are dishonorable only if they also harm someone else. But telling lies that are self-serving and harmful to others can never be construed as acceptable behavior. I recognize that dishonest behavior has degrees of guilt and accountability associated with it. There is a difference between "stretching the truth" about whether your spouse looks as if they are putting on weight versus lying about cheating on an examination, for example.

Surely most of us exhibit dishonest behavior from time to time, but all of us must work to be honest in all that we do. I admit that I have been dishonest at times, and my dishonest behavior is perhaps the greatest source of regret that I have in my life. I recognize that I am imperfect, as all of us are at times, but I am committed to be honest and honorable moving forward. I hope I will be setting the proper example for my children and their children as well as anyone else whose behavior I influence. I hope that reading this book will have a positive impact on readers, including my family, as they consider their own behavior when honesty is a difficult choice. I also hope that my family will come to understand how I think and behave better than they did before I decided to share my thoughts in this fashion.

Now, let me tell you about Christine. I first met Christine in the operating room (OR) at Long Beach Memorial Hospital. She was under anesthesia, so she cannot say that she met me at the same time. I had been in my office across the street from the hospital seeing patients when I received a call from the OR. One of the OB/GYN doctors was operating on a 55-year-old woman with a uterine cancer. His assistant was his office partner. Most uterine cancers are early stage. A simple hysterectomy is often sufficient management for many such patients. He assumed that would be the case in scheduling her operation, so he didn't send her to me for surgical management. He had removed the uterus in which the cancer was located without complication and had the pathologist evaluate the specimen by taking a frozen section of the uterus. Frozen sections are often used as a means of determining a diagnosis during surgery when the diagnosis is uncertain. Frozen sections are also employed frequently when a cancer diagnosis is known, but additional information from the pathologist during surgery can influence the extent of surgery that should be performed. The pathologist found that the cancer had spread from the uterus down into the cervix (stage II), which meant that the operation which had consisted of a hysterectomy with removal of the uterus and ovaries and tubes was incomplete. The lymph nodes needed to be removed to determine if there had been further spread. OB/GYN doctors are not trained to do lymphadenectomies (complete removal of the lymph nodes in the pelvis and lower abdomen), so he called me to complete the operation.

We performed this operation around 1995 at which time the best incision for this procedure was vertical (up and down from the pubic region to the umbilicus or even higher). This incision permitted easy removal of the lymph nodes, when necessary. This was prior to the era of minimally invasive surgery done with a laparoscope or robotic assistance using multiple tiny incisions in the abdomen. Minimally invasive surgery permits safe removal of the uterus, ovaries, tubes and lymph nodes with improved cosmetic result and a quicker recovery than with a vertical incision.

Because this doctor didn't anticipate the need to remove lymph nodes, he had made a low transverse incision (bikini incision) for cosmetic reasons. This was not the best incision for me now because the lymph nodes are higher up in the abdomen than the uterus, ovaries and tubes and I needed to remove the lymph nodes in the pelvis and along the lower portion of the aorta. So, I called for my fellow to assist me. He came over from the office so we could remove the lymph nodes together. His assistance helped assure optimal exposure that permitted safe removal of those lymph nodes. Meanwhile the other two OB/GYN doctors left the OR and went back to their office.

Now I should mention, that when surgery is performed in the abdomen or pelvis it is common to use sponges, or more properly bulky sterile cloths to hold tissues out of the field of surgery and permit its safe performance. Those laparotomy pads, referred to as "laps," might or might not be completely visible to the surgeon while performing the operation. The prior two surgeons had placed several "laps" in the abdomen. They were not easy to see. While I was there, I also placed some "laps" to improve exposure of the region where the lymph nodes were located and permit the safe removal of the lymph nodes. I proceeded to remove the lymph nodes, as required, and then I left the OR for my fellow to close the abdomen. I had to return to my office which was full of patients awaiting my return.

My fellow, had not been present at the start of the operation, when the two other surgeons were operating. He arrived after I first started working on the lymph nodes. When I departed my fellow commenced closing the abdomen. When he was done, he returned to the office to assist me there. As always, the nurses counted the "laps" as the surgery was ending and reported the "lap count" at the completion of surgery as correct.

Christine stayed in the hospital a few days longer than usual but was doing well. I counseled her that she would need radiation therapy to reduce the risk of cancer recurrence in the pelvis since the cancer had spread to the cervix. Her lymph nodes were not affected by the cancer which meant that her prognosis for cure was excellent. She was fine with the plan for radiation treatments and went home in about a week. Over the next few months, she required a couple of admissions for fevers that I could not explain. I treated her with antibiotics. She would get better and go home and then come back again a few weeks later with the same complaints. Meanwhile I was unable to administer her radiation therapy because of her recurrent infections. Radiation therapy in the presence of an active infection can cause serious complications. Furthermore, she had severe rheumatoid arthritis being treated with methotrexate, and was quite uncomfortable since she could not resume her arthritis treatments because of the fevers. Finally, after several months we obtained

X-rays of the abdomen and pelvis and saw a bulky soft tissue mass in the pelvis on the images.

I took Christine back to surgery and found five "laps" in the abdomen which I removed. How is that even remotely possible? First you must understand that there are nurses who assist the surgeon(s) in the operating room. There are the circulating nurses who are responsible for anything that occurs away from the operating table . Among other responsibilities, the circulating nurses provide "laps" to the scrub nurse who in turn hands them to the surgeon when requested. The scrub nurse assists at surgery by supplying instruments, sutures, "laps," etc. as needed by the surgeon. The "laps" are handed from the circulating nurse to the scrub nurse in groups of five. This is done for ease of tracking them during the operation and confirming that all of the "laps" have been removed from the patient's body at the end of the operation.

So here is the problem. When the circulating nurses counted "laps" at the end of an operation 25 years ago at this hospital, they didn't count the actual number of laps that had been given to the scrub nurse , they only counted groups of five "laps." As an example, if the scrub nurse was given 20 "laps" during the course of an operation, (that would be five "laps" given at four different times during the course of the operation), the circulating nurse would group them in fives's at the end of the operation after all of the "laps" were believed to have been removed. If their count showed groups of five's to be complete, the count was reported as correct. So, they didn't actually count 20 "laps" in this example, they counted four groups of five. In fact, if there was a missing "lap" they would come up with three groups of five laps" and one group of four. The circulating nurse would report an incorrect "lap" count and the surgeon would know one was missing and still in the patient. The surgeon would search until that fifth "lap" was recovered. No one had ever lost five "laps," so there had never been a need to count the total number of "laps" before. In this case with Christine, we didn't start the operation, the exposure was limited by the poor choice of incision by the OB/GYN doctors and my fellow, who closed the abdomen, wasn't there when the "laps" were put in the abdomen. Furthermore, he did not look very hard to find any of them because the circulating nurse provided a correct "lap" count. There might have been 20 "laps" used during this operation (four groups of five) but only 15 "laps" were retrieved (three groups of five). There you go, five laps left in the abdomen. Needless to say, practice now is to count the total number of "laps" rather than just groups of fives in the OR at this hospital!

Now just to clarify what might be confusing, not all "laps" are placed inside the abdomen such that they would be out of the sight of the surgeon. Most are actually used to remove blood from the operative field or otherwise facilitate exposure without the need to leave them in the abdomen for any period of time. Under most circumstances, only two or three laps are actually placed inside the abdomen for much of the procedure such that they are at risk to be unseen as the operation is being completed.

Unintentional leaving "laps" behind does occur from time to time because of an incorrect count by the circulating nurse. Typically, these occurrences require additional surgery and usually result in malpractice suits that are loved by patient's attorneys since they invariably result in a large payout to the patient (plaintiff). This payout, referred to as "damages" is to compensate the patient for her pain, suffering, out of pocket costs, anticipated future costs for possible additional care, etc. The nurse's error inevitably falls on the shoulders of the surgeon and the hospital which employs the nurse (defendants in the malpractice case). The surgeon is often referred to as the "captain of the ship." And when a ship sinks, it is the responsibility of the captain to go down with the ship.

I guess it would have been possible to hide this information from Christine and just say that I had found an infection or some other explanation for the need for additional surgery. However, I took responsibility. As soon as Christine awakened, I told her what had happened and apologized for my error. I didn't blame my fellow or the nurses or the other surgeons. I simply owned up to the error. As the surgeon at the completion of her cancer operation it was my responsibility.

I had the hospital's risk management team talk to her. They offered her some money. She was grateful the mystery was solved, and that the cancer had not recurred. Now she could go back on her medications for rheumatoid arthritis. I never did start the radiation therapy because I was concerned that the adhesions in the pelvis from the "laps" would put her at high risk for complications with therapy. So, she was happy about that. She did accept the hospital's offer of money and never contacted an attorney.

I wish the story ended there, but a year or so later she came back in the hospital with a bowel blockage which was directly related to adhesions caused by those "laps" we had left behind. After trying to manage her without surgery it became obvious that she would need an operation to correct the problem. When I offered having another doctor do the operation, she would have none of it. I guess she figured no one would be more careful than I would in taking her back to surgery with what happened the first time. Furthermore, she really liked me as her doctor. I had been honest with her; I had apologized and was contrite. She valued my honesty and the care I had given her, so I took her to surgery and corrected the blockage. She did fine thereafter. I continued to see her in follow up until I retired, nearly 25 years after her first operation. We always had a good laugh about it when she came in to see me over the many years that she has remained cancer free.

CHAPTER EIGHTEEN

DISCIPLINE AND PATIENCE

CYNDI

This book is all about self-betterment. One of its goals is to encourage introspection. I hope it invites readers to look in the mirror and see their strengths and weaknesses. The anecdotes I present are often interesting and thought provoking, but the real goal here is to make ourselves better, kinder, happier and more forgiving beings. All of us are extraordinary in many ways, but sometimes it is easy to overlook who we are and more importantly, who we can be.

Two additional important personal aspirations that are intertwined and, at times, confused with each other are discipline and patience. Let me try to distinguish these two important qualities.

Discipline is maintaining a commitment to study, read, observe, and prepare, over what typically is a long time for the purpose of achieving an important goal. A helpful tool to achieve discipline is passion, because discipline typically requires strong motivation. Passion fuels motivation. I was passionate about becoming a physician and having the opportunity to care for sick people long before I decided to become a gynecologic oncologist. That passion provided the motivation to study hard for the years required to become a physician. I became so very disciplined when it came to deciding between partying or studying.

I have observed that many very bright high school students are motivated to become physicians. However, when they get to college and enjoy college life, fraternity or sorority, partying, etc., they no longer have the discipline to focus on study at the expense of self-gratification. Long term goals become subordinate to short term gratification. Studying to be a physician or a lawyer or any other line of skilled work requires discipline. Therefore, discipline typically requires both time and great effort. The goal of discipline is achievement as measured by reaching important personal goals.

Patience is the willingness to wait to accomplish a goal. Discipline requires patience because most important goals are achieved after great effort over a long period of time. Patience does not necessarily require discipline, however. A willingness to postpone starting a family or vacationing in Italy might be important decisions; however, they do not require discipline. No special effort is required to postpone desired personal wishes or goals. Let me give an example that illustrates how discipline and patience are codependent when making treatment decisions on many patients with cancers. It took me many years to achieve my goal of becoming first a physician and then a gynecologic oncologist. That required a lot of learning, preparation and focus, while missing gratification that might have come earlier from other pursuits that I could have achieved with less effort. In other words, it required discipline to become a gynecologic oncologist. As a gynecologic oncologist I learned through study and observation how cancers grow and how they respond to treatments, such as chemotherapy and radiation therapy. Those patterns of growth enabled me to patiently await treatment responses before making further recommendations for some of my patients. Accordingly, patience created opportunities for me that might not be afforded the impatient physician. Practicing patience, in this example, is a passive act requiring first observation and second, decision-making. But just imagine the discipline required to reach this critical decision making in my career.

Not everyone has had the discipline or motivation or passion to become a physician or an attorney or an electrician, for example. In the broader sense, however, self-control requires discipline. All of us should exercise the discipline necessary to maintain self-control in our interactions with others. It is accomplished through time and effort with a focus on the achievement of an important personal goal. Thus, achieving self-control meets the criteria for exhibiting discipline. The important goal is self-betterment through impulse control.

Self-control requires a pattern of behavior that is respectful and not offensive. Threats to self-control must be avoided. For example, alcohol or other psychoactive drugs such as "marijuana" inhibit normal impulses and can result in a loss of self-control. I would never respond to inflammatory emails or texts after having a drink or two, because I knew my message might damage relationships through a loss of control caused by the alcohol. I offer these suggestions through the window of many years of interpersonal interactions, not all of which were as kind and respectful as they should have been, especially after enjoying some wine or bourbon or perhaps a martini or two.

This introduction gives me the opportunity to tell you about Cyndi who was in her 40s when she was sent to me in the early 1990s with a newly-diagnosed cervical cancer. She was a successful accountant employed by one of the "Big Five" accountancy firms. After her cancer diagnosis, her firm released a few of their junior employees. She was one of them. She was understandably upset without a job and expiring health insurance. She had initiated litigation against her firm for "wrongful termination" which she believed was because of her cancer diagnosis. In California, a state known for its robust employee protections, fired employees still rarely can sue an employer for wrongful termination successfully. Nevertheless, Cyndi successfully litigated a wrongful termination claim and won a large settlement from her company after completing treatment for her cancer.

My evaluation of Cyndi showed that the extent of her cancer precluded surgical management. She would be treated best with a combination of radiation therapy and chemotherapy with the drug Cis-platin. She understood that her ovaries would be destroyed by the radiation and that she would need to go on hormonal therapy. My examination showed that the cancer had grown onto the right pelvic wall to which it was attached. She had pain in the right hip, probably from the cancer putting pressure on nerves in that region of the pelvis. To this day I can recall the physical findings on Cyndi's pelvic exam. We call that stage III-B with an expected cure rate of about 50%. I recommended therapy consisting of radiation treatments five days a week for six weeks along with six weekly chemotherapy treatments, all of which she tolerated well. The radiation therapist followed this external beam radiation with two additional courses of internal radiation called brachytherapy. The goal was to maximize the dose of radiation delivered to the cervical tumor and tissues around the cervix including the vagina, uterus and parametrial tissues (those tissues that surround the cervix). The expected response was a gradual reduction in the size of the cancer with what hopefully would be its complete destruction. Tumor reduction is measured by physical examinations every few weeks beginning about two months after completion of therapy.

When I first examined Cyndi two months after completion of therapy, there had been little measurable response to the treatment. Sometimes response to therapy can be delayed, but I was concerned by the lack of a response early on. I suggested that I see her every two weeks to evaluate her response and she agreed. Over the next six to eight weeks there was little response which was very worrisome, and I shared that information with her. I also began to discuss a possible surgical approach if the tumor persisted. Unfortunately, in this circumstance the surgical procedure would require removal of the bladder, rectum and vagina if I was going to be able to offer her the possibility of surgical cure. I would need to create a colostomy for her plus a new bladder constructed from a portion of her intestine. Even with such an extensive operation, the probability of cure would have been no more than about 50% if surgery was required.

Cyndi was young and was willing to undergo anything necessary to save her life, so she was on board. And then, two weeks later, for the first time, the tumor was a bit smaller by my physical examination. And two weeks after that, still smaller until about six weeks later, I could no longer feel evidence for remaining cancer. We had been incredibly patient, beyond the point where we could have reasonably expected her to have been cured by her radiation and chemotherapy, but now there was no measurable tumor. I had her undergo needle biopsies into the area where the cancer had been located with the aid of CT guidance. The biopsies were negative for tumor. They showed only the characteristic pathologic effects of the radiation treatments. This was the hoped-for result of therapy.

Cyndi has done well for the past 25 years without recurrence of her cancer. With the rather large settlement from her accounting firm, she was able to move to Florida, where she lives in the Orlando area. She keeps in touch with me every year on her birthday by email to let me know she is fine. I did see her one more time when I was in Florida, when I traveled with my wife, Marlene, for a meeting of the Society of Gynecologic Oncology. Cyndi looked and felt great. She was and continues to work as a realtor, never getting back into accounting. She is healthy and happy. She is a testament to the value of good clinical judgement and patience borne from the lessons I learned while training to care for women with cancers such as Cyndi's. Discipline resulting in anxious patience was a winner once again.

CHAPTER NINETEEN

THINKING OUTSIDE THE BOX
DUYEN

What does it mean to "think outside the box?" It is a popular phrase, but what does it really mean? It is another means of saying "be creative," to try something new that others have not and typically would not do in a similar circumstance. Rules and traditional thinking need to be discarded and novel thinking must be adopted.

The world of medicine in most circumstances is orderly and treatment options are well documented for most medical conditions. Best treatments ideally are determined through rigorous scientific investigation. During the global coronavirus pandemic in the 2020s, we heard about Phase III studies of COVID-19 vaccines to determine the best way to protect the population from the deadly virus. These Phase III studies typically compare one treatment option (or vaccine for example) with another one in which the goal is to determine which option provides a better outcome for the condition being treated.

Phase III clinical trials typically are designed such that patients are randomized as to the treatment they will receive (It is like flipping a coin to decide which of two treatments will be administered). Furthermore, ideally neither the patient nor the doctor knows what treatment is being given. This is referred to as a "double blind" study.

It is actually very important that patients be randomized into one of the treatment options to avoid investigator bias or patient bias into the study. Studies in which patients are not randomized often provide inconclusive results to the investigating physician.

Let me offer an example to show how that works. Suppose the *New York Times* publishes an article about an exciting new drug (let's call it "Superdrug") for advanced pancreatic cancers where two patients at UCI Medical center who were believed to be incurable have had a remarkable response to this treatment for three years. There is even the possibility of cure for what otherwise is viewed as an incurable disease. There is another treatment for pancreatic cancers that typically is used for similar patients that sometimes provides a remarkable response that can last for over three years. That other treatment represents the standard treatment for this devastating disease. So, the investigators decide to compare the standard treatment with Superdrug. Now the doctors that enroll patients into this study are really excited about Superdrug even though it is unclear if it is more effective and less toxic than the standard treatment. Two remarkable responses do not justify changing established therapy that has benefited some patients previously. So, let's assume that two patients who are eligible for the study present to one of the investigating doctors. One has much less spread of the cancer, is younger and stronger than the other one. The doctor knows that a patient with less disease, is younger and stronger than another has a better chance of a good response to any treatment, so he/she is motivated to put the more favorable patient on Superdrug. The doctor knows that the other less favorable patient has a lower chance of a great response to Superdrug because that is the natural history of cancers. Less favorable patients based on cancer characteristics and personal performance usually do less well than more favorable patients. The doctor is very excited about Superdrug and wants it to have the best chance of performing better than the standard treatment. If the patients are randomized to receive either Superdrug or standard treatment, the doctor's bias preferring to administer Superdrug to the more favorable patient is eliminated. If, on the other hand, the doctor can choose which patients get Superdrug and which do not, more favorable patients will selectively get Superdrug and Superdrug will outperform standard treatment. But in this case, better performance of Superdrug would result from patient selection by the doctor rather than being a more effective treatment.

Perhaps more confusing is the importance of performing double blind studies in which neither the patient nor the doctor knows which treatment is being administered. With the example above, the patient may have read or been told about this exciting new treatment. The patient really wants to go on Superdrug, but it is only available to patients on a study. So, if the patient is told that he/she is randomized for standard treatment, there is a risk that the patient will decide to drop off the study since the motivation to be on the study was a chance to receive Superdrug. Likewise, the physician has a strong motivation for his/her more favorable patients to be on Superdrug. If the doctor is aware that such a patient does not randomize to Superdrug, there is a greater risk that the physician will take the patient off study for a variety of reasons such as moderate toxicity that otherwise would be viewed as acceptable if the patient was on Superdrug. When patients drop off study for reasons such as these, the data analysis at completion of the study can be compromised and the results suspect. The bottom line is that patients on Phase III studies must be treated the same regardless of treatment selection and that is less likely to occur if either the patient or the doctor is aware of the treatment.

There are Phase III studies of cancer treatments, hypertension, diabetes, hospital acquired infections, and so on. Even the management of hip fractures, bleeding complications of surgery, or heart attacks are subjects of clinical investigation. Investigation through Phase III controlled clinical trials with randomization of patients provides the gold standard for establishing best treatments for a given condition.

But not all diseases lend themselves to such studies, especially those that are very rare including some cancers. Likewise, when the clinical condition is difficult to document such as fibromyalgia or whiplash injuries, clinical trials have been difficult to perform. And sometimes very rare diseases present with an even rarer clinical scenario, where the usual treatments have failed and all will be lost unless "thinking outside the box" wins the day.

Such a condition occurred with a Vietnamese patient. I'll call her Duyen. Duyen was 33 years old when I met her at my office at the UCI Medical Center. She had undergone a supracervical hysterectomy (the cervix was not removed) by an OB/GYN in Fountain Valley for excessive uterine bleeding. This had caused her to become anemic. It is unclear why he did not remove the cervix; however, it is an easier operation to leave the cervix behind rather than removing it when performing a hysterectomy. Nowadays, OB/GYN physicians do supracervical hysterectomies much more frequently than complete hysterectomies which include removal of the cervix. It is an easier operation, so that is the usual reason it is done that way. The surgeon did not identify a cause for the bleeding. Only after the pathologist reported a choriocarcinoma in the uterus was the cause obvious.

As an aside, in my autobiography, I had written about my invitation to join the Public Health Service to serve as my military obligation during the Vietnam War. That invitation came from Dr. Roy Hertz at the National Institutes of Health (NIH). One of his major accomplishments there had been the discovery of drug treatment for choriocarcinoma, a fast-growing cancer, that had spread to the lungs in three women who were dying of the disease. (The drug was

Methotrexate. It's also used to treat cancers and other diseases. For example, my wife Marlene and thousands of other rheumatoid arthritis patients have been treated with Methotrexate over the decades). His treatment was the first ever successful drug treatment of a cancer and established chemotherapeutics as a means of cancer treatment and possible cure. All three of Dr. Hertz' patients were cured with methotrexate. By the way, this is one example in which treatment of only three patients completely changed therapy for this previously incurable cancer.

When I saw Duyen, the diagnosis of choriocarcinoma was known from the pathologist's evaluation of the uterus. The appropriate studies included measuring the pregnancy hormone, human chorionic gonadotropin (hCG) which is normally produced by the placenta of a normal pregnancy, but in this case was produced by the cancer cells. Since her uterus had been removed, I knew that the elevated hCG was not due to a pregnancy. Her level was elevated indicating that there was still cancer present in her body. I also ordered several scans to see if there was any evidence for spread of her cancer. There was none. As she was not cured with the hysterectomy, I started her on a course of the same chemotherapy that Dr. Hertz had administered in the 1950s to his patients at the NIH. I would know if her cancer had responded by a change in the hCG levels. When levels become undetectable, the patient usually is considered cured. If the levels do not go to zero, she is not cured. It is a simple yet elegant test for this rare malignancy. There are no other cancers for which a simple blood test reliably predicts a high probability of cancer cure with treatment than choriocarcinoma.

Duyen initially had a decrease in her hCG but it didn't go to zero. Furthermore, she continued bleeding suggesting that she likely had more cancer in the cervix that had not been removed during her first operation. I operated to remove the cervix, which did, in fact, contain cancer. I restarted her on another chemotherapy drug. Between the surgery and the second drug, her hCG levels fell to zero. I expected that she was cured, because about 98% of patients whose hCG drops to zero with treatment are cured.

I continued to follow Duyen with measurements of hCG monthly for about a year, at which time her levels began to rise. This meant that there was cancer elsewhere in her body. I ordered scans to locate the areas of spread, but they were negative. I knew there was cancer present because of the rising hCG levels; however, the amount of cancer was too small to show up on any scans. At that point I started her on an intensive chemotherapy regimen of three drugs, a part of the standard treatment of such unusual patients. As expected, her hCG levels dropped to zero. I was confident that she was finally cured. About a year later, however, her hCG levels began to rise a second time, so I restarted an intensive multidrug regimen that is typically used in this circumstance. Once again, after a few months of treatment, her levels fell to zero, but I was less convinced that she was cured, based on her history.

After about eight months her hCG levels began to rise again. At this point there were no clear cut guidelines about treatment. I repeated her scans, which were negative, but I knew that there was disease somewhere. The most likely area was the lungs, but the most sensitive scans including CT and PET scans failed to show any disease there or elsewhere. The amount of cancer in Duyen's body was simply too small to be seen on any scans. I started her on a newer biological agent but her hCG levels continued to rise. Again, the scans were negative, but I was confident that the cancer was in one or both lungs, since statistically that was the most likely area of spread.

At that point, most physicians would continue to try different chemotherapy regimens since these cancers typically respond well to these drugs. But she had convinced me that she had a resistant area of cancer that we were unable to find and that was unlikely to respond to any other chemotherapy drugs. So, I decided to wait and watch, rather than treat her further. I waited as her hCG levels began to rise, month after month. Finally, after about three or four months, the hCG levels had risen to a level where I thought another scan might reveal the location of the resistant disease. In other words, I had intentionally given the cancer cells enough time to start growing up to a point where the cancer would be visible on scans. Sure enough, a small area on one of the lungs, measuring about a half inch in diameter showed up for the first time. I was elated. I was confident that this was her cancer and I believed it was her only remaining cancer that we had not been able to eradicate.

I contacted our cardiothoracic surgeons and asked them to remove the area of lung that had showed up on the recent scan. They were hesitant to operate on her because cancers that spread to the lungs are almost never curable with surgery. I told him that this was an exception, that if he removed the growth in the lung, I was confident she would be cured. He was more than skeptical, especially since there were several lymph nodes in the lungs that were also enlarged on her scans. He thought they were probably areas of cancer as well. I told him that these cancers rarely went to lymph nodes, and while I didn't know why they were enlarged, I didn't think it was from this cancer. With my insistence, they took Duyen to surgery. Surgeons found the small mass and removed it, and it contained choriocarcinoma. They also removed the enlarged lymph nodes, which tested completely normal.

I have lost contact but Duyen remained disease-free for three years after her surgery and is likely cured. This was an exercise that required patience, self-confidence, a profound knowledge of the enemy (the cancer), and a willingness to think outside the box. The reward was the cure of a young woman with a long life ahead for her.

CHAPTER TWENTY

IMPORTANCE OF TEACHING

LUISA

For many years, beginning in the late 1980s until 2005, I traveled as often as monthly to Las Vegas to train residents there and operate on many of their most complicated gynecologic oncology patients. For three of those years beginning in 1997, I worked extensively with one of the residents, Dr. Mark Turner, who was interested in becoming a well-trained pelvic surgeon performing the same kinds of operations that I did. His goal and that of the chairman of the Dept. of Obstetrics and Gynecology, Dr. Joseph Rojas, Sr., was for him to be able to provide the surgical care needed for their patients with gynecologic cancers in my absence.

The assumption was that the medical oncologists in Las Vegas would continue to administer the chemotherapy for these women just as they did when I operated on them. Since gynecologic oncologists typically administer chemotherapy to their patients, Dr Turner would not be a trained gynecologic oncologist, rather a well-trained pelvic surgeon. In other words, Dr Rojas was looking for a way to replace me there with Dr. Turner so that urgent cases could be operated on without depending on my scheduled visits. I was more than willing to help.

I always enjoyed going to Las Vegas; however, I was not a gambler and not particularly interested in the night life or the entertainment. Furthermore, I had plenty of clinical, teaching, and administrative work to do at UCI Medical Center, even though I really did enjoy working with the Las Vegas residents as well. I should mention that during the years that I operated in Las Vegas, there were no gynecologic oncologists in the city, so I was the only game in town for several years. Emergencies that arose in my absence and cases that simply could not wait until I was scheduled to return usually were managed by OB/GYN's along with general surgeons.

Now let me share my observations about operating with OB/GYN residents as compared with post residency fellows training to become gynecologic oncologists. I have always been committed to training fellows to become excellent gynecologic oncologists and leaders in the specialty. I have also always loved working with residents, especially in the operating room. Frankly, it takes intensive surgical training of fellows over at least two years, performing hundreds of complicated pelvic and abdominal operations to produce a competent gynecologic oncologist. I loved doing it. Training post residency fellows who would become gynecologic oncologists while caring for women with cancers were my primary goals during my long career. Still, operating with OB/GYN residents six or eight times while on the gynecologic oncology service can make a tremendous difference in developing their surgical skills which they can rely on for the remainder of their careers. Performing a few hysterectomies with residents teaches them valuable surgical skills they will use going forward while caring for their own patients. I know this is true based on so many unsolicited notes from former residents.

In the early years while I was at UCI, faculty would be evaluated annually by the residents. That is a valuable exercise which permits faculty to see how trainees view the teaching abilities of their mentors.

Every year, virtually every resident who rotated on the gyn/oncology service commented on the value of their surgical experience when operating with me. Ninety minutes in the operating room performing a hysterectomy with a resident paid much higher dividends for that resident than a single operation performed with a fellow did for the aspiring gynecologic oncologist. During such operations I could teach residents how to apply my four laws of surgery while helping them improve their surgical skills

As one might expect, even as an itinerant physician coming and spending a day or two operating in Las Vegas with the residents each month, I still had the opportunity to make a difference in the lives of some of those patients. One such patient, (I'll call her Luisa) sent me a card in 1997 that read:

> Some things we will own forever, the memory of the just, the remembrance of a good act, the good remembrance of someone fair. This will never be taken from us. This we will never give away. (This marvelous sentiment was based on a Mexican Nahuatl Indian Song).

The 27-year-old woman who sent me this card also wrote a very nice personal note to me just prior to Thanksgiving and a few months after I had operated on her with Dr. Turner for a pelvic mass that proved to be an ovarian cancer. She expressed gratitude that I had rearranged my schedule at the Las Vegas clinic so I could operate on her. She said she was surprised that I would do that for her since I really didn't know her. She was grateful that "you took over 45 minutes reviewing my lab slides and never billed me." It is funny that not billing her was important to her and contributed to making me a special physician in her mind. She enclosed a small gift, a music tape for me to listen to. She had listened to it often the summer after her cancer surgery.

Its message gave her peace. She said:

> I think you will find it quite interesting since you are a physician that really cares about your patients. Have a very Happy Thanksgiving. I know I will. I have a lot to be thankful for this year.
>
> Gratefully, Luisa

She enclosed a photo of her with her young daughter, Lauren, 2 years old, holding onto her neck and showing a big smile with four baby teeth. I do not recall the message in the tape which I did listen to, but I do remember this special young lady who had an early-stage ovarian cancer. I hope she is doing well.

Looking back on my career, I love that I was able to make a difference in the lives of my own patients. But actually, I know that I also made a difference in the lives of hundreds and even thousands of women who were cared for by the physicians that I trained. Those physicians were delivering the care that my colleagues and I taught them, in the clinic, by the bedside and in the operating room. It is a measure of paying it forward for the training I received as a fellow decades ago. Impacting the lives of thousands of women directly by my care and indirectly from the care provided by my former fellows is the most important professional accomplishment of my life.

CHAPTER TWENTY-ONE

FAITH AND PRAYER : CAIS

Luisa's story reminds me just how important hope, prayer, and faith are when having to face a serious illness such as a cancer. Many of us who rarely if ever pray will rely on prayer and find renewed faith if we face a cancer diagnosis or some other life-threatening illness. Prayer provides comfort for the patient as well as loved ones. I think prayer is one of the most important coping mechanisms we have to deal with life's most difficult events—tragedy, illness, death, etc.

The concern of our cancer patients, of course, is not only for their own wellbeing, but also for that of loved ones left behind. Luisa had a 2-year-old daughter around whom her world revolved at the time of her cancer diagnosis. Facing her own mortality at this time seemed unfathomable. Even patients with a profound faith who do not admit to a fear of death, still grieve when considering their own mortality because of the impact on those they will leave behind. I've noticed this wish to survive is strongest among those with small children. That observation is not to diminish the desire to live which exists among all of us when facing a similar circumstance.

Life is precious and what happens after we die will always remain a mystery. The unknown is unsettling. And yet, when quality of life is irreversibly poor, patients often will welcome their own passing. All of us come to understand that our time on Earth is limited and that someday all we hold dear and all earthly possessions will no longer matter. So, our goal should be to live a healthy and a long life that is also a life full of goodness. All of us want to be remembered by those we leave behind as loving, kind, and charitable in word and deed. That should be our legacy. There is simply too little time to waste on making bad decisions and missing opportunities to do good.

I don't have stories of bad decisions made in the care of my patients, even though undoubtedly there must have been some. Some might call that selective amnesia. Perhaps that is the explanation. I also do not have stories of lives wasted because of poor choices. But I would like to share a story of a woman with young children who had an incurable cancer, although at this time she is still alive. We will call her Cais, who is Vietnamese.

Let me begin by stating that the presentation and behavior of cancers usually exhibit a high degree of predictability. For example, ovarian cancers spread throughout the abdomen and respond predictably to specific drugs. Cervical cancers rarely spread as ovarian cancers do and tend to grow locally within the pelvis without spread for many months and sometimes for years. When spread occurs, typically it is to lymph nodes in an organized fashion. It is this predictability of the behavior and response of cancers that permits a rational approach to its treatment. Ovarian cancers spread throughout the abdomen, so we remove as much as we can surgically and then we use chemotherapy drugs that are well standardized. The success of the operation and the effectiveness of the chemotherapy will determine whether a patient will be cured or how long a patient is likely to live if not curable. Advancements in ovarian cancer treatment, especially with newer agents such as PARP inhibitors (targeted cancer drugs) and anti-angiogenic agents for example, have resulted in prolongation of life for many such patients, but cure rates remain poor. In contrast, cervical cancers remain localized for a long time in most patients, so localized therapy, either surgery or radiation treatments combined with chemotherapy often offer the best results.

Sometimes, however, the only predictability of a cancer is how unpredictable it can be. For example, sometimes drugs that usually will not benefit an ovarian cancer patient work beautifully and at times drugs that usually work very well will not be of benefit. Once we understand the hows and whys of this unpredictability, we will be on our way to curing many more patients who have this lethal disease. The answer will lie in continued advancements in understanding cancer genetics and the ability to modify those genes responsible for cancer development.

Cais was sent to me around 2012 with an advanced ovarian cancer. Most ovarian cancers are advanced when diagnosed as I have observed previously. I managed Cais in the usual fashion, with an extensive operation in which I removed as much of the cancer as could be removed safely and then administered six courses of the standard chemotherapy. I started her on Carboplatin and Taxol every three weeks.

Taxol was originally found and extracted from the needles and bark of the Pacific Yew tree. It was very expensive when first produced because of the costs of production and the limited geographical distribution of the Pacific Yew. It is a lot cheaper now that it is synthesized in the lab and also because the patent for its distribution expired many years ago.

In any case, Cais began therapy within three weeks of her operation and received six courses in the standard manner over a total of four months. Her CA-125, which had been markedly elevated at the time of her diagnosis, fell into the normal range, as expected. Except for the total baldness and mild numbness in her fingers, Cais did well. There was no evidence of any remaining cancer at that time.

The usual schedule of follow up after completion of chemotherapy is at three-month intervals for two years and, if disease free, at four to six months thereafter. On those occasions she was evaluated with physical examinations and CA-125 measurements. Cais did well for about two years after which her CA-125 began to rise. This change was a reliable indicator that her cancer had recurred. We say it recurred, but in reality, it was never completely gone. Perhaps we should say the cancer resurfaced since it was there all along, but we didn't have clinical evidence of it. When there is no evidence of a cancer following treatment, it is "in remission." Unfortunately, remission does not equate with cure. Even if we had a crystal ball that told us with certainty that there was still cancer present, there would have been no benefit of restarting treatment earlier than when it became obvious that she was not cured.

You will recall that I mentioned previously that we used to do "second look" operations to determine if there was still any cancer present after the chemotherapy. The information gleaned at this second operation didn't improve patient outcome. In other words, knowing there was still cancer present sooner than was evident on exam or CA-125 measurements and then restarting chemotherapy earlier than clinically indicated, gave the same results as just waiting until there was clinical evidence such as a rising CA-125 or a mass found on exam, before restarting chemotherapy.

I explained about the need to resume chemotherapy to Cais when her CA-125 began to rise. She was understandably saddened but agreeable. Afterall, at that time she had two daughters, one in middle school and one in high school. She wanted to see them grow into adulthood. Since she had done well for two years it seemed reasonable to restart a chemotherapy regimen that was similar to the Carboplatin and Taxol. I did make an exception, however, since she had experienced some numbness in her fingers with the first chemotherapy which is a side effect of Taxol. Worsening numbness was likely if I restarted the Taxol. This would likely cause permanent nerve damage in her fingers and toes. Worsening nerve damage in the fingers might eliminate sensitivity to touch, high temperature and pain sensation. This effect, called neuropathy, can even affect sensation in the feet when walking. That is an unacceptable side effect, so I started her back on Cisplatin, which is related to Carboplatin, along with another drug, Gemzar. It turns out that she did great on this combination of drugs. By four months of treatment her CA-125 was normal and she felt fine.

I should mention that Cais is a stoic person, as is her husband. But they were understandably elated. I knew, however, that this journey was not over. Ovarian cancers that recur once almost always continue to recur until the patient dies of her cancer. There was no reason to share that information then. I joined them in their happiness. Sure enough, a year later her CA-125 began to rise. I started her on a different chemotherapy regimen which was ineffective. The standard is to avoid treatments given previously if a cancer recurs within a year, so initially I didn't want to restart the same drugs; however, when the new drug was ineffective, I had nothing to lose so I restarted the platinum agent with Gemzar. Surprisingly, she had another complete response to therapy and did well for another year.

One year later, she became symptomatic for the first time, so I needed to treat her to relieve her abdominal pain and fluid in her abdomen which was compromising her quality of life. So, I restarted the same two drugs, and once again she had a marvelous response with disappearance of her pain and abdominal fluid. Her CA-125 which was initially elevated returned to normal.

This cycle continued annually for a total of five different cycles of these drugs. Each time the therapy put her into remission, meaning no evidence of cancer. There were times when we tried other newer drugs on a clinical trial, but that never worked. Each time we went back to the same platinum plus Gemzar with a good response every time. The final time I treated her, the response was much less robust and durable, so around the time that I retired in 2018, we were trying other newer treatments. At that point I said my goodbyes to her as I did to all my patients.

In October 2020, I was thinking about Cais, so I contacted one of the fellows at UCI, Diana, and inquired about my former patient. I was thinking she had probably died. I really cared about Cais, her strength, her faith, her humility, and her will to live. It turned out that she was still alive but having more problems from the cancer. She had recently been hospitalized for a bowel blockage. She was being discharged and had been recommended to go on hospice for comfort measures. Coincidentally, that's when Cais contacted me, since she had my email address. I had given my email address to many of my patients prior to my retirement. I wanted them to know that they were important to me and that I was available for them if they wanted to contact me. Several actually have contacted me for a variety of reasons, some related to their cancers, some for another medical issue and some just to keep connected with me. Cais told me what I had already learned from Diana and thanked me for giving her eight years of life.

Cais was grateful to be able to see her children grow to adulthood. She had no regrets despite the difficult effects of the cancer and its treatment on her life and that of her family. The good times far outweighed the bad times for Cais. She told me that she was not finished yet and that she wanted to try to live a little longer. She asked for my advice, so I suggested that they try that same chemotherapy regimen for a sixth time. I felt there was little to lose. It had been two years since she had received these drugs. I shared my recommendation with Diana who passed it on to her current physician who agreed with my plan.

I know that Cais was still alive as of January 2021, and she and her daughters continue to keep in touch with me. She sent me a very nice note at Christmastime with a thoughtful gift. Her faith is strong and she believes in the healing properties of prayer. This belief system has carried her through many difficult years with hope and without despair.

CHAPTER TWENTY-TWO

FEAR AND VULNERABILITY

CASSANDRA

When I began writing this book, I wanted to explain what has been most important to me during my professional life. With this purpose in mind, I've shared stories about some of the patients I have cared for over the years. I also wanted to share how I became the person I have become over the past 80+ years. It has not been a perfect life, but hopefully it has been one in which my imperfections have been offset by a lot of hard work, a genuine commitment to providing the best possible care to women with cancers, a love of teaching, and a life full of compassion, honesty, love, kindness and gratitude.

I also wanted to share some of the stories of these amazing women who entrusted me with their lives to illustrate their strength and resilience when facing a cancer diagnosis. Their trust in me is the most humbling demonstration of confidence, faith and love that I can imagine. When we drive over a bridge, we do not usually think of the engineer that made it safe to do so. When we enter a building, we do not often think of the architect that designed it. When we take an antibiotic for an infection, we do not think of the laboratory that discovered it. But when physicians accept responsibility for making life and death decisions for their patients and managing their care, their acts are remembered and replayed by our patients and their loved ones throughout their lives. That is the impact that physicians have, especially those of us who care for the sickest patients. Our actions are transformative for their lives and those of their loved ones.

Medicine is not a profession for those who are unwilling to work hard, because the preparation for and practice of medicine is difficult. I also believe that medicine is not for those who cannot make a lifelong commitment to the betterment of their fellows, or those who lack in self-confidence, or those who are self-centered. But medicine is the most noble of pursuits for those who choose that honorable profession. In this chapter and the ones that follow, I would like to share some more stories of patients who, through the years, became my friends as I cared for them at vulnerable times in their lives.

I recall the first time I met Cassandra in 1984. Both she and her husband were attorneys. Her husband had been a college standout on the gridiron. He had been drafted by an NFL team in the first round. He subsequently was traded to a team I followed. Then he went to law school and worked as an Assistant US Attorney. While Cassandra was under my care, he provided me memorabilia after I told him I was a lifelong fan. I never told him that I didn't remember him on the team.

Cassandra had also gone to law school and was an attorney when she met and married her husband. She has a daughter who graduated *magna cum laude* and later, from law school. This was a seriously smart and take-charge kind of family. They very much liked to be in control of their lives, but this situation was not in their playbook.

Cassandra was diagnosed with a cervical cancer. My exam showed the cancer was early and measured no more than two centimeters.

These are highly curable with either surgery or radiation therapy combined with chemotherapy, with a cure rate of about 90% for either approach. I discussed these two options and specifically recommended surgery. She was only in her 30s. I would save her ovaries with surgery since the cancer was confined just to the cervix. Furthermore, surgery would likely avoid the risks of radiation therapy which would include destroying her ovaries, possibly causing long term adverse effects on her intestinal function and occasionally leg swelling from the scarring that radiation produces in the pelvis. Cassandra was agreeable, and I performed the indicated operation without complication a couple of weeks after her initial evaluation.

Cassandra was a worrier. She tended to see a glass as half empty rather than half full. If there was a 90% of cure, that meant to her that there was a 10% probability of her dying from her cancer. That knowledge was incredibly unsettling, so she wanted to improve her odds. She wanted me to administer radiation therapy as well, even though she was likely cured and even though adding radiation therapy would only add to the risk of complications without adding to her likelihood of cure. It took months for her to get past this thought process and typically it took long office visits to reassure her and help her get past her fears. I am not certain that she ever got past that fear completely.

Now, to make things more difficult, several months after her operation there were subtle findings on her pelvic exam that I noted and mentioned to her. In hindsight it might have been better to keep the information to myself; however, I always attempted to be honest with my patients, whether the news was good or bad. The physical findings felt like scarring to me which can occur following surgery. I explained that such changes were not too uncommon and that I was not concerned that her cancer had recurred. I planned to monitor it with periodic exams. She would have none of it and insisted on additional testing to be certain that the cancer had not returned. So, I acquiesced and ordered a CT scan. It was normal. I reassured her, but she would have none of that either, so I ordered an MRI scan, which was also normal. She continued to ask for radiation therapy, and I continued to dissuade her. This went on for many years after her operation, during which the cancer did not recur. She was fine physically but an emotional wreck. Her problem was that she was a pessimist and a worrier and was never completely comfortable with her excellent but not perfect prognosis. This woman was accustomed to perfection, not merely excellence.

Whenever I saw Cassandra, I would provide reassurance to her about her cancer and later about personal issues that arose in her life. I might say, for example, that I was confident that her son would get into the college of his choice or that her daughter would pass the California bar exam. That reassurance was always followed with the same response, as if she were saying it cleverly for the first time: "From your lips to God's ears." I have often wondered if God actually has ears; however, I don't think she meant it literally. But it was so predictable, that when I would go in to see her during a routine follow up exam, I would bring in a medical student or a resident with the task to see how long it will take her to say, "From your lips to God's ears." Cassandra never let me down although on one occasion I was literally walking out the door of the office after the exam before she finally said, "From your lips to God's ears." I left the room and turned to the student and said, when *you* practice medicine, I hope you know your patients as well as I know mine.

The story has a good ending in that Cassandra's cancer never recurred. I saw her up to a few months prior to my retirement. She was fine and grateful for all the care and reassurance over the years. There had been one other unfortunate occurrence over the years. I had chosen surgery in part because it rarely causes leg swelling whereas radiation therapy does so more frequently. Cassandra did develop leg swelling in one leg as a very late complication of the surgery I had done, and over several years the swelling became quite severe. She did a lot of research on this, as I had expected, and came across various treatment approaches that she tried unsuccessfully. But she was o.k. with this, because she finally seemed to accept that she was cured of her cancer. She viewed the leg swelling as just the cost to save her life. And I guess, that is just what it was.

Certainly, most patients experience worry and doubt when first diagnosed with a cancer. Their fears usually dissipate with time, especially if they are doing well. This is an important coping mechanism that permits us to go about the business of living our lives in the face of uncertainty. It is the ability to accept uncertainty as a reality of life and to tolerate external as well as internal stresses. Patients such as Cassandra are able to cope less well than most others. Her fears undoubtedly diminished joy in her life as she faced them daily for many years.

Some patients can express their uncertainty eloquently when confronted with a cancer diagnosis. I received such a note dated September 2012 from one of my patients who was a nurse. She wrote it on awakening a few days after her doctor called her on the phone to tell her she had a rare form of uterine cancer.

The note was entitled "Cancer."

> "I was stuffing a turkey when the phone rang. I thought it odd to see the name of my doctor on the caller ID. I'd had a biopsy the day before and was told I would receive the results in a week. My doctor was pretty sure it was fibroids. So, I thought so too.
>
> [The doctor] is not only my gynecologist but my work colleague and friend. She spoke in a matter-of-fact way using the type of formal language usually

> reserved for the delivery of disturbing news. Hers was the same voice I use to tell a pregnant woman her baby no longer has a heartbeat.
>
> You have a rare form of endometrial cancer...I wanted to say 'what?' or 'really?' but I knew I had heard her correctly. As I hung up, I stared at the sticky clumps of turkey stuffing smearing the face of the phone. And then I lost my taste for turkey forever.
>
> I began walking in figure eights around the kitchen island and into the living room. (ever wonder why they call it a living room?) I felt unexplainably giddy and buoyant. I'm guessing this is healthy denial. My breathing was fast and shallow. It was as if I had floated up to a corner of the ceiling and was viewing myself from a different perspective. I have cancer?
>
> For several days I would wake up in the morning and there would be one precious moment....and then the remembering would come. There was a heaviness inside and when I got out of bed, I felt like I had left some part of me buried in the sheets. Then I would listen carefully. If I could hear one bird singing, then I knew everything would be okay. I started to wonder what makes birds sing but, really, I don't even want to know."

This is a heartfelt note from a woman dealing with a new cancer diagnosis. It probably expresses feelings experienced by so many of my patients over the years. Early in the note there is the acknowledgement of the possibility of dying. "Why do they call it a living room...as if I had floated up to a corner of the ceiling?" is a description from people who have experienced near death events. And then, she expresses hope in the form of a bird. "If I could hear one bird singing, then I knew everything would be okay." And finally, when she says, "I don't even want to know," she is expressing the feeling that she does not want to know the outcome of her pending journey, accepting the uncertainty of her future. What an emotional roller coaster, written so eloquently. I must say that I do not recall this patient very clearly, but I will never forget the note she sent me to share her fear, her vulnerability and her wish for a cure.

If you have never experienced a life-threatening diagnosis and if all your family members and friends are in good health, it might be difficult to relate directly to this story. Even so, it is difficult to avoid feeling empathy for her. How would you react to a friend or colleague who was like my patient? Would you feel awkward and be unable to offer comfort? Would you feel discomfort in her presence and avoid her? Imagine yourself in a similar situation and ask yourself what you would hope to hear from your friends. You would probably hope for friendship, love, compassion and companionship. Remember, it is always better to say something than ignoring the reality of the moment.

CHAPTER TWENTY-THREE

UNINTENDED CONSEQUENCES
MEG

There are times when patients or their families make decisions that are unwise, often against advice. They can have dire consequences. Inevitably they are always made with the best intentions, but the outcome can be disastrous. I would like to share with you one such event.

I remember well my octogenarian patient, Meg, who was sent to me in the 1990s with an aggressive uterine cancer. She was probably 83 or 84 years old at the time of her referral to me. She lived in Palm Springs, California with her husband of more than 50 years. They were a very cute and loving couple. I enjoyed the opportunity to care for her. Uterine cancers are usually managed initially with surgery which is the complete treatment for most such patients. Some, however, are at high risk to recur and additional therapy can be indicated. As I have discussed previously, further treatment can consist of radiation therapy or chemotherapy depending on the surgical and pathological findings. Widespread cancer requires chemotherapy while cancer confined to the pelvis at risk to recur in the pelvis is often treated best with radiation therapy.

Meg had a cancer that seemed to be confined to the uterus, but microscopically appeared to be very aggressive. For a younger woman I would likely have recommended both radiation therapy and chemotherapy after surgery; however, that seemed too aggressive for such an elderly woman. A frail, elderly body often will not tolerate surgery plus radiation therapy plus chemotherapy. Accordingly, I operated on her successfully and without complication. After six weeks I recommended a course of radiation therapy to the pelvis since I believed that was the most likely area to which the cancer might spread. I thought this would give her the best chance of cure.

Radiation therapy administered to the pelvis is usually tolerated well, even by elderly or infirm patients. Meg tolerated it without difficulty. Early side effects such as diarrhea usually are managed easily with modification of diet and the administration of antidiarrheal medications such as Imodium. Unfortunately, delayed complications of radiation can include damage to the intestines. This occurs in less than 10% of such patients. If the damage causes a blockage to the rectum or lower colon a colostomy might be indicated. If the damage is to the small intestine, which is much more common, medical management is best. Only in the most severe instances is surgical correction recommended for radiation damage to the small intestine. Meg developed characteristic symptoms and X-ray finding of small intestinal damage from the radiation about 18 months after receiving it. Her symptoms were nausea, vomiting, abdominal distension, and abdominal pain.

Meg came into the emergency room with these complaints. After an examination and some abdominal X-rays to confirm the diagnosis, she was admitted to the hospital. The usual treatment of bedrest, intravenous fluids and no food or medications by mouth (nil per os, nothing by mouth, NPO) was initiated. Within two or three days her pain, nausea and vomiting had subsided. We began to feed her.

First, we gave her clear liquids and over a couple of days advanced her to solid food. Before discharging her, we discussed dietary measures of multiple small meals daily of well-cooked foods with low fiber content to reduce the probability of a recurrence of symptoms. Then she went home back to Palm Springs.

It would have been nice if this were the only such episode; however, it happened again about a year later. Again, admission, bed rest, NPO, IVs, slow progression of diet over several days, and then discharge to home. The guidelines for surgical management were and continued to be inability to maintain nutrition, intractable pain not relieved by conservative measures or blockage of the small intestine not relieved by these measures. Meg didn't meet the criteria for surgery, so she was treated "conservatively" as described.

Now I wish that these were the only two such episodes, but they happened several times, maybe four or even five with the same outcome each time. She was always able to be sent home after five or six days in the hospital. They occurred about once a year. It was distressing for her and her husband and it was distressing for me as well. But she was getting the appropriate care and she was not a good candidate for surgery. Surgery in the face of radiation damage to the small intestine is risky with the potential for serious complications. It is not likely that Meg would survive a serious complication of surgery for intestinal damage from radiation therapy.

One day, some family members came to Palm Springs, perhaps on a vacation, or perhaps just to visit. They noted that the Mayo Clinic in Scottsdale, Arizona had a wonderful reputation and was only a four-hour drive from Palm Springs. They wondered if a second opinion about her care at the Mayo Clinic would be a good idea. Meg was about 89 years old at this time, had all her faculties, and she wanted to please her family. So, Meg's family called the Mayo clinic and made an appointment for her to see one of the gastroenterologists there in consultation. She didn't see one of their gynecologic oncologists, which likely would have been a better choice. In any case, Meg was seen, her history was taken carefully, X-rays were reviewed, and the gastroenterologist decided that he was uncertain if this was a problem with the small intestine or with the colon. He should have known better, but apparently, he wanted to be sure that he knew just what was going on. He suggested that Meg undergo a colonoscopy to see if the colon was responsible for her recurring problems (it was not, by the way). So, Meg had an appointment made to come back a few days later after undergoing the needed bowel prep for colonoscopy, which she did. The colonoscopy was complicated by a perforation of the bowel. This was not a big surprise to me when I learned of it, since the colon was also damaged by the radiation therapy, even though that was not the cause of her symptoms. Radiation damage to the colon subjects it to an increased risk of perforation with colonoscopy. Meg died four days later from the infection that followed her colon perforation.

I do not know if there is really a moral to this story or some hidden message. It is a sad one with a terrible and unnecessary outcome. I learned of this event from a copy of her records from the clinic where the colonoscopy was performed.

I guess one message is that, if a patient would like another opinion when complications of therapy occur, it would be best to discuss it with the treating physician, especially if you have confidence in that physician. And I guess, if you are a family member of such a patient, it might be best to express your concerns to the patient but leave the decisions to the doctor and the patient. Imagine the guilt felt by the family and the heartache suffered by her loving husband. I guess the overarching message is that life is not fair and there should be no expectation of fairness. Just enjoy the good times and do not be surprised when the bad times come along, as they inevitably will.

CHAPTER TWENTY-FOUR

GRACE AND SPIRITUALITY
SISTER MONICA AND BARBARA

I love when patients are gracious and spiritual in their interactions with their healthcare providers, especially when I am that provider. It should come as no surprise that some of the most memorable occurrences have come from members of the clergy that I have cared for over the years. They really know how to be spiritual and express their gratitude and show grace. Furthermore, as far as we can know, they might even have the ear of God at their disposal.

I took care of two nuns at different times, both at Long Beach Memorial Hospital. Both were always extraordinarily grateful for my care and gracious to me. These two women were in convents when each was referred to me. Both had pelvic malignancies, and, as I recall, both were cured of their cancers with surgery and chemotherapy. Who knows, there might have been some divine intervention assuring their favorable outcomes. I do recall that their cancers were life threatening and how gracious they were after I had cared for them. I will mention one of them, Sister Monica, whom I treated in 2007. She sent me two notes, the first shortly after I operated on her and the second after five years of follow up, during which time, she was cancer free.

In a note dated August 2007, she wrote:

> Thank you for all you did to put me on the road to recovery. I don't have words to express how truly grateful I am... Please accept my promise of prayers for you and your loved ones. May God continue to enlighten and direct you in your efforts to bring healing to all those you serve.
>
> God bless you!
>
> Sr Monica.

Her note also read,

> Your kindness shines like the sun.

I like that simile a lot! Now, I for one, especially appreciate when a person of the cloth asks God to bless me and to help me bring healing to my patients. I hope God has listened to Sister Monica, because those were really important requests she sent to him on my behalf and for my patients. I'm just saying.

Her second note after it was clear that she was cured read as follows:

> I will always be grateful for who you are and for all you have done for me. While I look forward to returning to my community, I am sad that I have to say goodbye to you. I promise to remember you and pray for you always, in this life and in the next. I count on your prayers for me.
>
> With affection, Sr Monica.

I loved that she promised to keep me in her prayers. There is no greater gift that she could have offered me. And I have kept her in my thoughts and prayers over the years. I gladly welcome such wishes from persons of all religions because you just never know when God is listening or to whom He is listening.

I believe that spirituality should be an important part of our lives. I spoke of it briefly in an earlier chapter. It provides meaningful structure to our behavior. Without spirituality there is an empty place in our hearts. Spiritual people, in my experience, deal better with serious adversity than those who do not have a strong belief system. As much as anything else in life, spirituality provides comfort for the dying. Spirituality permits the dying to understand that "Death is not the opposite of life, but a part of it" said Haruki Murakami, who is a famous Japanese writer. It is our destiny. A belief in a God offers the promise of a companion on our final journey. I believe in God although I have no preconceived sense of a hereafter. As a practicing Jew, there is much ambiguity about the afterlife. If there is an afterlife, I just hope it includes bagels and cream cheese with lox. I guess I will see eventually, or maybe not.

I think I have had only one patient who thought of me as a friend first and her doctor second. That is Barbara. She was certainly on the autism spectrum and was domiciled in assisted living after her father died a few years before I met her and became her doctor. She had lived with him for the first 40 years of her life. Social services arranged for her assisted living arrangements after he passed. Barbara was pretty independent in that she could get to my office using public transportation and then return to her domicile without assistance, but she could not live independently. She was a unique individual in many ways. For example, she was a calendar savant. If you told her your birthday, she could quickly tell you the day of the week you were born. The first day we met she asked me my birthday and in a couple of seconds told me I was born on a Wednesday. I checked. She was correct. She loved showing off this skill since the feedback was always so positive. Whenever she came into the office, I would introduce her to a student or resident who accompanied me into the examination room, and then she would ask him or her the date and year of birth. Quickly, my charge would know what day of the week that occurred. Some would go back to the office and look it up. She was never wrong.

Barbara was difficult to miss when she came in to see me. She had a loud booming voice that always announced her arrival. As soon as she was checked in, I knew that Barbara had arrived. When she saw me, she always said, "Hi Dr. Berman," as she was being weighed or having her blood pressure checked. Whenever she left the office, she remembered to say, "Thank you Dr. Berman." If it was around the time of a holiday, she always greeted me with Happy Hanukkah or Happy Passover or whatever. She also liked sending me cards around the holidays. Hanukkah was her favorite. Her cards usually were written for "A special friend."

On one such card she wrote:

> Dear Dr. Berman, It is a pleasure having you as my doctor and I pray that you and your family have a good Hananikah. [She was not a good speller]. You make me feel very good and I look forward to my appointments. Shaloh [I think she meant Shalom],
>
> Your patient, Barbara.

On the four-year anniversary of her operation that I shall tell about shortly, she sent me a Hanukkah card that read:

> Like latkes without applesauce or dreidels that won't spin, like menorahs without candles or like gelt that you can't win...Like Maccabees without their leader, Judah, brave and true, some things just wouldn't be the same without someone like you!
>
> Your patient, Barbara.

Barbara was a very simple soul and extraordinarily loveable.

I met Barbara after she had been admitted to Long Beach Memorial Hospital with heavy vaginal bleeding. She was in her mid-40s. The first thing she told me was that her father had died. No expression of sadness, only a matter of fact, "My father died." I had not even asked her, but it was on her mind and she always spoke whatever was on her mind. I learned that she had heavy vaginal bleeding and was anemic.

Her admitting doctor had found a mass on her cervix. She told me so. I examined her and biopsied the mass which was a cancer. Under the microscope it was characteristic of a uterine cancer, so it appeared that she had a cancer that started in the lining of the uterus and grew down to involve the cervix. We call that Stage II.

I told Barbara that she needed an operation to remove the cancer and her response was "All right doctor." No questions, no comments, no concerns, just "All right doctor." So, I did a hysterectomy to remove the cancer and took additional biopsies of lymph nodes to see if there was evidence for spread of the cancer. There was none. Because of the involvement of the cervix, I recommended radiation therapy after she recovered from her operation to reduce the risk of a cancer recurrence in the pelvic region. As expected, she said "All right doctor" and "Thank you doctor." So, she had radiation therapy without difficulty and was fine for several years. That note she sent me at the four-year mark after surgery she wrote:

> Dear Dr. Berman, Happy Hanukkah (she got the spelling right this time) to a good surgeon. You are proof that your patients are feeling good and that includes me. It is four years now. Look forward to my next appointment. Barbara.

Unfortunately, her cancer recurred in the pelvis despite her radiation therapy, probably six or seven years after her initial surgery, which was quite unusual. Most often these cancers will recur within two to three years when they do recur. She never had any questions about the recurrence or my recommendations for chemotherapy. When the chemotherapy didn't help much, she developed a colon blockage which required a colostomy. When I prepared her for the surgery, she said "All right doctor" and "Thank you doctor" and then I operated on her. She was fine with the colostomy and named it "Dr. Berman" since I had done the surgery. It made perfect sense to her. She learned how to manage the colostomy by herself being able to empty the colostomy bag of waste and change the bag when indicated. I thought that was pretty amazing, as it is not an easy task to master. As her cancer progressed, she became weaker and weaker but never complaining, and always "All right doctor" and "Thank you doctor." Even when I told her that she was dying her affect didn't change and she just accepted it without question. I do recall her saying that she was going to see her father, and I said that was right. She was fine with that and always agreeable and grateful.

Sometimes life is not fair, as all of us know, and this was certainly the case with Barbara. I probably have thought about Barbara after her passing more than most of my other patients. There is a saying that I think Barbara would have spoken if she had wanted to comment before her passing. "Fear of death is ridiculous, because as long as you are not dead you are alive, and when you are dead there is nothing more to worry about." She just never expressed any concern and, even though I never thought of her as especially spiritual, I think she welcomed the chance to visit with her father once again. Well, dear Barbara no longer has anything to worry about except the sadness that her passing created for all of us who cared for her.

CHAPTER TWENTY-FIVE

OTHER STORIES

Sometimes patients "fire" their doctors. When they do so, usually they just do not return for a scheduled follow-up appointment and instead go to a different doctor for their subsequent care. They do not usually call and say "Doctor, you're fired." I know that all doctors have some patients that have fired them. I am no exception even though I do not have certain patients that come to mind when I think about this subject. But I am reminded that, from time to time, I have fired patients from my practice and told them that they cannot come back to see me. Whenever that happens it is critical to recommend other doctors they can see to provide for their care. Otherwise, I could be charged with abandoning my patient. That would be a very bad thing to do with potential legal consequences. So, providing follow up with another doctor is critical, especially if a serious diagnosis such as a cancer is present. When the diagnosis is not serious, as in a patient who has no cancer or other life-threatening disease, the need to provide follow up with another physician is necessary but less problematic.

You're Fired! When I decided to write about firing patients, a few of them came to mind. Do not get me wrong, I very rarely did this, and always for what I considered to be a valid reason. For example, I had a patient from the south that accused my fellow, a black physician from Alabama, of improperly touching her during his examination. I knew that he would never do such a thing. He had examined hundreds of patients for me during his fellowship without a single complaint or concern. I also confirmed that he did the examination with a chaperone in the room and there were no issues or patient objections that arose during the exam. (A chaperone should be present during any examination in which the patient is undressed for a breast and/or pelvic examination. This is true even when a female physician is examining another woman, in my opinion). I discussed her claim with the patient who was adamant. I believed that she was simply a racist and was offended at being examined by a black physician. I told her that she could continue to see me in the future until such time that she found another physician to provide for her care, and in any case, no longer than three months. I gave her names of several doctors she might want to contact for follow up. She was fired!

I had another patient who had fibroids and was unhappy about them even though she was not symptomatic. There really was no compelling reason for me to be following her since she did not have cancer; however, she was pleasant and wanted to see me. I have always been a softie for such patients over the years and had a number of patients with benign conditions who just liked the way I spoke with them and provided for their care. I saw this young lady on several occasions during which she expressed a wish to have the fibroids removed and during which I told her there was no reason to do so. She had no pain or bleeding which are the typical indications for surgery in such patients. Rarely fibroids are removed when they are thought to be a cause of infertility; however, she was not interested in becoming pregnant when she was under my care or in the future. She disappeared from my practice for about six months and then came back to see me after undergoing a hysterectomy performed by another physician. She liked me much more than that surgeon, so she wanted me to continue providing her follow-up care. I fired her! If she had had cancer and if the operating physician was inconvenient for her follow up, I would have continued to take care of her, but this was inexcusable behavior to me. I encouraged her to return to the operating physician for follow up.

One of the more interesting cases was a woman with a cervical cancer I had treated with radiation therapy and chemotherapy. She had stage III-B disease which is quite advanced, but was treated successfully with chemotherapy and radiation therapy. She did well but wanted to sue the doctor, a pathologist, who had caused a long delay in establishing her cancer diagnosis. I used to do a lot of medical malpractice consulting, so when her attorney asked me to be a paid expert on her behalf, I agreed to do so. I felt that she had been injured and deserved compensation. (If I write a third book, undoubtedly it will be a compilation of medical malpractice cases I worked on with innumerable attorneys over the past 30 years.) The proof that she had a long delay in her diagnosis was from her Pap smear that had been misread. If it had been read properly, the cancer would have been diagnosed more than a year earlier. That long delay resulted in progression of her cancer to a more advanced stage with a poorer prognosis and fewer treatment options.

The attorney sent her Pap smear slides to me to aid in my evaluation of the claim against the pathologist. Somehow those slides were misplaced by office personnel and never found. The misread slides would have provided the proof that the pathologist was responsible for the delay in diagnosis, so, loss of the slides meant that the malpractice case was lost for my patient. She sued me and was awarded some money from my malpractice carrier. I do not recall how much money was awarded, but it was not a huge amount.

Then she came back to see me because she wanted me to continue being her doctor. I gave her the names of other local gynecologic oncologists and then I fired her! I cannot say that I blame her for following her attorney's advice to sue me; however, I just didn't feel that I had a continued obligation to care for her.

Time is a resource. The last case I would like to share is a patient that came within a hair of being fired; however, I warned her about this possibility, but never actually fired her. We will call her Roberta, who was about 50 years old when she was referred to me with a newly diagnosed uterine cancer. It was high grade which meant that her prognosis was uncertain and that the risk of advanced stage or a later cancer recurrence was high. Her only fault was that she was so high maintenance, and she had a daughter who was even more difficult to deal with than she was. Each visit was 45 minutes or longer, always reviewing issues we had discussed previously. And then her daughter would come in and would want to review the same issues again. We discussed her disease, staging of cancers, the role of surgery and radiation treatments, prognosis, risks and benefits of therapy as I did with all my patients. But no matter how much time I spent with her and her daughter, it never seemed to be enough for them. Finally, I remember saying that I was not sure that I was the best doctor to be taking care of her because I just could not devote as much time with them as they expected. I suggested that I could send Roberta to another excellent doctor who would provide the care she deserved and, hopefully, meet all her expectations.

That little pep talk was all that seemed to be required. Afterwards, Roberta never brought her daughter with her to the office and she agreed to all my recommendations. Our subsequent meetings were typically 10 or 15 minutes which is appropriate for follow-up visits. I did her operation and recommended radiation therapy which she underwent without problems. For many years afterwards she came into the office for her follow-up appointments and never expressed any concerns.

Roberta disappeared from my practice for a few years as she was cured and did not really need my follow up. Then one day my office took a call from her asking that I come to see her. She had been admitted to a local community hospital with a bowel obstruction. The surgeons there who had seen her in consultation at the request of her admitting doctor were planning to operate on her for this. The bowel blockage was likely related to scarring from the radiation therapy she had received while under my care. Her story was almost identical to Meg's who died following an ill-advised colonoscopy that I shared previously. Roberta wanted to know what I recommended.

I went to see Roberta later that day and outlined a conservative, non-surgical plan of management which I hoped would avoid surgery. This was the same plan of management that I outlined in Meg's care previously. The doctors there did what I recommended, and she was discharged without needing surgery several days later. Roberta sent me a nice note a few weeks after discharge which read:

> Dr. Berman, I want to thank you for seeing me at Los Alamitos Hospital. You made it so easy to know what to do. It took them a while to get the plan, but we finally got it right. I appreciate having such a great doctor!
>
> Sincerely, Roberta.

She returned to my office for regular checkups after that hospitalization and never had further intestinal problems. I saw her last just a few months prior to my retirement and at least 15 years after her initial treatment. I do not think there is an important message in this case, but it was interesting, and the outcome was good, so I thought I would just share it. It is still hard to believe that general surgeons would take the advice of a gynecologic surgeon in the management of a bowel obstruction. But they did and the patient benefitted from it.

The Bikini Cut. At times I have modified the surgical management of some of my patients to meet their needs or expectations. One classic example is the surgical approach to the women with cervical cancers. For several years of my career, my usual surgical approach was done through a vertical incision from the pubic region up to and even around the umbilicus. This always left a rather large scar. Even though I would carefully close the wound as cosmetically as possible, younger patients hated the scar. There was no way for them to wear a bikini after this type of surgery because the scar would be visible. Bikinis are a big deal in Southern California where the sun always shines, beautiful bodies without ugly scars are treasured, and the ocean beckons.

After a few years I began offering a low transverse incision (bikini cut) to the thinner patients for cosmetic regions. By being thinner I could accomplish all that was necessary through this more attractive incision. The only problem was that it required more room than was afforded by the usual bikini cut, so I had to cut through the abdominal muscles to gain sufficient exposure to perform the proper operation. That meant no six-pack abdomens for these young women. The cut muscles would never be as strong, even after healing, as they had been prior to the operation.

Then one day a 30-year-old with an early-stage cervical cancer came in for me to care for. I discussed the choices of an up and down incision. She was horrified. I discussed the possibility of a bikini cut but warned that by cutting the abdominal muscles she likely would have poor muscle tone and a bit of a pot belly. She was dismayed at that possibility as well. She looked at me, batted her eyelashes and she pouted. She actually pouted. Finally, I offered a similar operation with a bikini cut but without cutting the muscles. Instead, I would remove the attachment of the muscles to the pubic bone to give me room to do the correct operation. Then I would reattach the tendons of the abdominal muscles to the pubic bone when I was done. I had not done that before for patients with cervical cancers but was pretty sure that it would work fine. So that is precisely what I did, and it worked like a charm. She was cured of her cancer and had a beautiful flat abdomen, much to her delight. Whenever she came back to see me over the next several years, she always asked if I still did the special operation I had devised for her on my young women with cervical cancers. I was able to answer her honestly that I did.

While I certainly didn't invent this incision (It's called a Cherney incision reported first by Leonid Cherney in 1943, the year after I was born), I think I refined it a bit for the purpose of the radical hysterectomy. The patients liked it a lot, especially in the light of the necessity to have an operation to cure a cancer. At the same time, I did develop and refine some other surgical procedures that other physicians have adopted over the years. For example, I developed a means of creating a tunnel for a catheter that had been placed through an abdominal incision into the bladder to avoid leakage of urine following removal of the catheter. In certain operations including some radical hysterectomies for cervical cancers it often is best to place the catheter into the bladder in this fashion.

I also developed a technique that avoided excessive blood loss while performing ultraradical pelvic operations. These techniques have been published and are a part of my contribution to the surgical specialty. I always loved the opportunity for creativity in the operating room.

Hey, is that you Dr. Berman? Occasionally I was able to interact with some of my patients outside the clinical environment. I always enjoyed seeing them, sometimes in Costco or at the REI store. I don't go to too many other stores except maybe Total Wine when my wine or bourbon stores are low, so those would be the most likely candidates. I recall seeing patients I recognized who were so used to seeing me in a white coat that they did not recognize me at first.

One patient whose story I would like to share whom I often saw outside of the office or hospital setting worked at a Greek restaurant I frequented over the years. My daughter, Vicki's, wedding rehearsal dinner before her wedding was held at this restaurant. My patient, Afra, was Iranian. She was an accomplished belly dancer. I always enjoyed her dancing at the restaurant, as well as, some fine Greek meals, especially the lamb chops. She had been referred to me with a uterine sarcoma which is another very aggressive type of cancer that can arise in the uterus. I had operated on her and had found spread to pelvic lymph nodes, so I had her undergo pelvic and aortic radiation therapy to minimize the risk of cancer recurrence. She did well for about five years without recurrent disease. She enjoyed life and was a lot of fun.

One day she came to see me at my office with abdominal pain. A scan showed evidence for recurrent cancer in the upper abdomen. I took her to surgery and removed as much cancer as I could remove. Surgery was very difficult, and I knew I had not removed all of it. That was impossible. I tried various treatments over the next year or two during which time it became clear that she was going to die. Her one wish was to get back to her home in Iran to visit her family. We sometimes use the term "tune up" in medicine as in automobile maintenance. You make some minor but necessary adjustments to the vehicle so it will run a little better and last a little longer.

Well, I tuned Afra up so she could return home. When she got to Iran, she sent me a warm note which read:

> Dear Dr. Berman,
>
> Thank you so much for giving me opportunity to visit Iran and my family. My flight even though was 22 hours, but it was very nice. I'm here right now four days and weather is not too cold yet. I'm going by train to Holly area in Mashhad north of Iran to pray for me and all sick people. My family and I leaving tonight. The city of Tehran is so crowded and very heavy traffic. If you are not a professional driver, there is no way you can drive here. It is worse than Italy. I usually call taxi come to my sister's house to take me wherever I need to go. Taxi in here is very inexpensive.
>
> I miss you all and love.
> Afra

I never saw Afra again as she stayed in Iran until her death a month later. I have vowed to take her advice and avoid Iran, not that I needed her to warn me. I do miss her smile and her joie de vie; such a beautiful and joyful woman. She was in her mid-60s when she died.

The end is near. I have received many special notes from patients who are dying but wanted to thank me for taking care of them. These notes are among my most prized possessions. I recall a particular 48-year-old woman I cared for from 1994 to 1997. We will call her Mona. She had a condition with a long name, pseudomyxoma peritonei. This arises from the ovaries but also can arise from the appendix in women and in men. When a pathologist sees a biopsy of this type of disease, it does not appear to be cancerous when studied under the microscope. Furthermore, it does not behave like a cancer because it never spreads to other organs through the lymph channels or the blood stream or invade tissues as cancers do. Despite the lack of typical cancerous behavior, it can be deadly.

In this condition the cells produce lots of slimy fluid and can attach to other surfaces such as the bowel, liver, stomach, and so forth.

It does not invade the tissues, but can create havoc, nonetheless. These cells attach to the intestines and cause repeated bowel blockages which often are not correctable because no areas of bowel are spared. Furthermore, they produce so much fluid that the patient always feels full and cannot nourish herself. In the end it can be just as lethal as any cancer, but strictly speaking is not a cancer at all. The usual best treatment is surgical and neither standard chemotherapy nor radiation is of any benefit. However, in recent years many patients have benefited from treating the abdomen with chemotherapy drugs to destroy some of these growths. This is called hyperthermic intrabdominal chemotherapy. That form of treatment did not exist while I was caring for Mona.

Mona had advanced pseudomyxoma peritonei when I first saw her. Her abdomen was very distended from the fluid it contained. I operated on her and removed the fluid and as many of the growths as I could. There were thousands of these "implants" all throughout the abdomen. She got some relief for a while. As is typical, however, the cells continued to grow and the abdominal fluid reaccumulated. Finally, when she was no longer able to eat because of the massive fluid in the abdomen and the bowel involvement, I put her on intravenous nutrition (TPN) to buy a little more time for her. She was quite young and had teenaged children. As the end approached, she sent me a special note just a couple of months before she died.

> Dear Dr. Berman. I want to give extra special thanks to you for prescribing the TPN as part of my everyday treatment. It has added much needed energy to my life and I'm so happy to be functioning at a better level than I was a few months ago. At least now I can be productive with my activities at home and for that, I am very grateful. And, while I'm at it, I thank you for being the outstanding doctor that you are. I've always felt that I'm getting the best treatment possible!
>
> And, I thank you. Sincerely, Mona.

With all that was going on in her life, unable to eat, facing impending death she found the time to be thankful and gracious. She was such a special woman with a heart full of kindness and gratitude.

Medical Television Shows. One thing I am so grateful for is that none of these patients or others in my practice that I can recall have second guessed my recommendations or their care in the hospital because of something they saw while watching a medical show on television. These shows often are unrealistic and therefore can created unrealistic expectations of their doctor or the hospital and its staff.

The most realistic medical TV shows reported by physicians are *Scrubs* and *House*. Among other things, they capture the interaction between attending physicians and trainees well and usually are medically accurate. Furthermore, nurses are shown doing things that nurses typically do and doctors are shown doing their thing. Doctors do not typically start IV's or inject medications, that is what nurses and IV teams do. You don't have doctors transporting patients from the emergency room (ER) to the operating room (OR), because transporting patients is done by the transportation services and patients rarely go directly from the ER to the OR. You don't have neurosurgeons doing abdominal surgery and family physicians operating on patients. You don't see psychiatrists in the operating room, even if they have cared for the patient's emotional needs. You don't typically have complicated diagnoses made in the ER because such patients require extensive diagnostic testing often in the hospital. You don't see toxicology tests of drugs reported shortly after blood has been drawn in the ER because even negative test results usually take at least a day, and positive tests may take several days or weeks. And you don't see medical oncologists administering radiotherapy to their cancer patients as I recently saw on an episode of *New Amsterdam*, a show that I will comment on further in a moment. Radiotherapy is done by radiation therapists in conjunction with their radiation physicists and techs. You do see everyone in the OR wearing a mask and every patient undergoing surgery covered with sterile drapes.

There are lots of shows that are notoriously inaccurate in their portrayal of care provided in a hospital and the roles of doctors and nurses and other hospital personnel in providing patient care. I do not watch these shows generally, because even though entertaining, I find the medical inaccuracies to be distracting for me. Two of the worst series cited by physicians and nurses are *Grey's Anatomy* and its spinoff Private Practice. One show I have been watching lately is *New Amsterdam.* My girlfriend, Bonnie, loves *New Amsterdam* for the drama and the interpersonal stories, but I have to constantly remind her that it is as far from the real practice of medicine and hospital culture as it could possibly be.

In recent episodes I saw doctors starting IVs, administering drugs, hanging blood for transfusions and taking an unwilling patient to the OR for an amputation without obtaining his consent (without even trying to debride the wound and save the leg with the help of antibiotics, which would be the appropriate treatment). There was also the ER resident who ignores the ER chairperson's orders to use imaging before inserting a central intravenous line and then is congratulated by this same physician for doing it successfully against her instructions. By the way, the chairperson and the resident are also hot lovers who make out in the hospital with some regularity! Meanwhile the hospital director derails hospital board meetings and is more interested in social issues in the community than running a hospital. You must wonder why they do not consult with a physician or a nurse before developing these shows. A little bit of reality certainly would not be harmful and might help prepare viewers should they require hospitalization or an ER visit.

I have started on this rant because non-medical viewers generally have no basis to distinguish reality from fantasy in the practice of medicine as seen on medical TV shows. Furthermore, these shows might create unrealistic expectations when the viewer becomes a consumer of care in the hospital. For example, viewers might have unrealistic expectations about recovery especially following serious trauma. They see effective resuscitation in most instances when cardiopulmonary resuscitation (CPR) is administered to moribund patients on television, yet only a small percentage of such patients actually survive and leave the hospital in good condition. On TV, heroic operations such as heart transplants or major cancer operations often show the patient a day later, awake, talking normally, sometimes not on IV's or other support. The reality is such patients after recent operations often are still on a respirator, typically are on strong narcotics for pain management resulting in sedation rather than animated dialogue, and typically are receiving intravenous fluids with a catheter in the bladder and drains in the surgery site. While the presentations on TV of such patients' courses are completely unrealistic, this can result in expectations for results that are impossible to duplicate.

CHAPTER TWENTY-SIX

BEYOND SIMPLE GRATITUDE
CHEN-SHU AND KITTY

This last section of my narrative is entitled "Beyond Simple Gratitude." A patient who gave me a special gift such as a new Bugatti or a Ferrari F60 or even a Porsche 918 Spyder would go into this section. But there were no such gifts. A patient who flew me on her private jet to her private island for a weekend vacation would surely go here, but there were no private jets or private islands as far as I recall. There was a patient in Pittsburgh who raised racehorses that competed in the Kentucky Derby. She invited me to her Derby party one spring day in 1979. I learned to make mint juleps, which I love. Her horse came in last. By the way, mint juleps are easy to make. You just need some good bourbon (I prefer Buffalo Trace or Woodford Reserve, although more recently I have really enjoyed Longbranch Bourbon made by Wild Turkey), shaved ice, fresh mint and powdered sugar. It has been the official drink of the Derby since 1938. Yummy, but no car or private jet so far.

The most generous gift came to me from the daughter, Hua, of a wealthy woman, Chen-Shu. Chen-Shu came to me from her doctor in Taiwan who had cared for her during the previous 5½ years. She was diagnosed with an advanced ovarian cancer, as were so many of my patients, and had undergone surgery and several different chemotherapy regimens before she came to see me in May 2003. Her doctors in Taiwan did not feel that they had anything more to offer her. Her cancer had recurred extensively in the abdomen including the liver and her quality of life was poor. Her family was desperate for her to live longer, if possible, so they brought her to California. They called me on my cell phone while I was at a local airport about to travel for a meeting I was planning to attend. My administrative assistant knew that I was always happy to speak with patients, even when traveling, and had given her my phone number. I took the call and agreed to see her when I returned a few days later.

When I met Chen-Shu for the first time, I learned from her daughter that she had lost a great deal of weight and was eating poorly. Her abdomen was distended with fluid and cancer and was tender to the touch. I reviewed the scans she brought with her that confirmed extensive involvement of cancer in the abdomen including the liver. I was not very optimistic about further chemotherapy because she had already been on all the usual drugs for recurrent cancer. This was several years prior to the development of newer targeted agents such as Bevacizumab and PARP inhibitors I discussed briefly in an earlier chapter. I thought surgery might be helpful in decreasing the volume of cancer and possibly preventing recurring abdominal fluid caused by the cancer, but I didn't feel comfortable removing the cancer that was present in the liver.

Accordingly, I sent Chen-Shu to see Dr. David Imagawa in consultation. Dave is an excellent oncologic surgeon with a special expertise in liver surgery. He had been the liver transplant surgeon at UCI in the past. Dave and I had operated together on several patients over the years. We have published our surgical experience working as a team on extraordinarily complicated cases. So, we agreed to operate on Chen-Shu in an effort to provide comfort for her and, hopefully, to prolong her life. We did take her to surgery and performed an extensive cancer resection with removal of much, although not all her cancer along with a portion of her liver. There was no way to accomplish complete cancer resection safely. She was elderly but recovered uneventfully. She and her daughter were immensely grateful for providing her a chance at a longer life.

When her daughter brought her mom to see me several weeks later for a postoperative visit, she handed me a card with a gift enclosed. The card dated 6/25/03 read:

> Dear Dr. Berman,
>
> We cannot express the gratitude and joy that is in our hearts. Even though this is your work, and you do this every day, nonetheless, you have touched our family's lives. Your generosity and professionalism even came through the first contact we had with you, when you called us while waiting for your flight at the airport, for an informal consultation. Every little deed you do is greatly appreciated by our family. We are immensely grateful for the successful surgery and for taking care of my much beloved mother, who has sacrificed everything for her family. (That is so characteristic of Chinese families to respect and revere their elders). Please accept this gift from our family with our deepest and sincerest thanks.
>
> Respectfully, Hua and Chen-Shu family.

Enclosed was a gift card for $1000 for Ermenegildo Zegna clothing. I knew that I should not accept the gift, but I did so anyway. To have refused would have been insulting to her and to her mother and it would have also made me very sad.

I went to this upscale store and learned that $1000 did not go as far as I might have expected. I did find a beautiful sport jacket with black slacks that I loved and purchased. This was 20 years ago, so you could actually buy a sport jacket with slacks for under $1000 at this upscale men's shop. I was thinner then so, while I still have the jacket and slacks, they do not quite fit right now. But they do provide a strong motivation for me to lose ten pounds. There was a little money left over from the gift, so I also bought a beautiful belt. I must admit, it was the finest clothing I had ever owned. The Italians really do know how to produce magnificent garments from the finest cloths.

Shortly thereafter, I saw Dave Imagawa who confided that he had also received the same gift and had made a similar purchase. He was complaining, however, because now he was unwilling to compromise in his wardrobe purchases moving forward and expected that his clothing allowance was going to skyrocket. For years thereafter, Dave continued to complain to me about that gift, but his wardrobe was fabulous.

As a postscript, I received another beautiful note of gratitude from my patient and her daughter three months later. In that note she thanked me again.

> ...for having the wisdom, courage and stamina to perform surgery on a patient with advanced disease so that our family can enjoy my mom's presence and generosity a little longer. Even though you do this day in and day out, for our family, it feels like a miracle...And, we just wanted to share this great feeling of joy, celebration, and life, and to express our thankfulness once again.
>
> With much respect and gratitude, Hua and Chen-Shu

We had many more interactions in the office over the next couple of years and then, finally, a note sent late in 2005:

> Thank you for treating my mom for the last 2½ years of her life. We all feel she got to live those two extra years because of you. In total, she lived eight years since her first diagnosis and surgery of ovarian cancer. Please know that all your hard work, and efforts really make a big difference...We feel you all are doing very sacred work and feel honored by you. Hua.

In oncology we can make a big difference for our patients and their families even when that difference is not the cure of a patient. It is a beautiful feeling to receive notes of gratitude from surviving family members after a patient has died.

Some of my patients have expressed their gratitude and affection by offering me gifts they created for me. I had a young patient who had a severe brain injury in an auto accident many years earlier. She had been bright and had a promising career before her accident, according to her older sister who always accompanied her to my office. I saw her for a mass that proved to be an early-stage cancer of the ovary that I easily cured with surgery. She did not require further treatment with chemotherapy. She continued to follow up with me for several years. Although all her potential for a bright future had been lost in a moment so many years earlier, she had learned to make soaps in various shapes and colors. Some of them were very fragrant. At times she would bring me the soaps she made as a gift for taking care of her. Her sister said she did it on her own without her sister's prompting. I never used the soaps but loved seeing them in my bathroom over the years. They kept me connected to this sweet young woman.

Several of my patients have crocheted wraps, scarfs, and blankets for me over the years. Most of them have been "adopted" by my daughters. Some still are in use at their homes. One such patient sent me a nice note on December 2002 that read:

> Dear Dr. Berman,
>
> We hope that you will enjoy this Afghan for years to come. Each stitch was crocheted with our deepest gratitude to you for getting us through our recent illness.
>
> Sincerely, Sarah
>
> P.S. Instructions for care are enclosed. Each stitch was crocheted with our deepest gratitude.

How could I express my thanks to her for her thoughtfulness that could compare with her heartfelt gift to me? Patients and family members often feel that a small gift given in gratitude is too insignificant to be of value to the recipient when offering thanks for saving a life or improving the quality of life for a patient. Those gifts, however, mean everything to the doctor who provided that care. They represent love and gratitude, much more cherished than the monetary compensation provided by an insurer.

Many other patients brought me gifts throughout the year, but especially during the holiday season. Around Christmas I could always anticipate See's Candy, pies, fruit cakes, fruit baskets, wine, bourbon and scotch, gift certificates, and more. Scotch somehow always was the preferred liquor from gift givers who had not asked me for my preference in alcoholic beverages. Bourbon came from those who had asked me, just in case you might be curious. Still, I always appreciated most the gifts that reflected the personal efforts of my patients and their families. I loved knowing that they were thinking of me with gratitude while working to make something I would enjoy, something that would make me happy.

The daughter of one of my patients had learned to make flower arrangements and made a beautiful one for me. She was grateful for the care I had provided her mother whom I had treated from 1995 to 1998. Her mom had died from ovarian cancer, but her daughter was grateful for the three years she and her sisters were able to spend with their mother after her diagnosis. She sent me a nice note February 1, 1999 on a card that read:

> Thank you, You always do the nicest things.
>
> Dear Dr. Berman, I was so impressed with you when you first operated on my mom three years ago. Also, with the second operation and the fact that

everyone at UCLA Cancer Center knew your name. You have an outstanding reputation in your field of ovarian cancer. As a surgeon, you are considered to be one of the best, if not the best! (She really loved me!) We were so lucky that FHP (her insurance was through Family Health Plan) felt inadequate to operate on my mom. You have let us see you a few Mondays ago when you were booked full. You signed the death certificate when we got you up in the middle of the night. You put up with all our panic, concern and finally our acceptance of a disease that we knew eventually would cause my mom to pass away. You also put up with my sister Kathy's questions, you know, the scientist. (She really did have lots of questions). Thank you for giving us our mom for an extra three years (relatively pain free too)! Thank you for your talent, and your heart. We appreciate you and will never forget you.

Sincerely Jennifer

P.S. I hope you like the flower arrangement I made for you. It is a hobby of mine. I am not professional at it.

Her daughter also sent me a letter written the same day by one of her sisters about her mom. It was a mixture of sadness, nostalgia, humor and joy. In the letter she alerted friends and family that her mom lay down on December 29, 1998, and never awakened. This was not unexpected as she had decided not to undergo additional treatments when her cancer presented itself again with a rapidly growing abdominal mass towards the end of her life. Her mom had expressed the wish not to go through a slow painful demise; "She wanted to go peacefully in her sleep." She observed "a most kind and loving God gave her this blessing." She thanked so many people who had loved and cared for her mom to whom she was so grateful. She closed by observing that her mom "was always confounded that she raised four daughters whose culinary prowess seemed limited to muffins, meatloaf and reservations." Finally, "Thank you all for being part of her life. As she said many times, 'I've had a lot of fun.' So have we."

That is not the end of the story for this family. I have taken care of two of the four daughters, each of whom required a hysterectomy for non-cancerous conditions. Their final written correspondence was sent to me July 21, 2004, 5½ years after their mom's passing. It was a Hallmark card that said:

> This world needs more people like you...more people who are willing to leave things a little better than they found them, to reach out with compassion...people who are willing to put all selfishness aside to do the good, right, kind thing. It will make a difference someday to someone.

The handwritten notes from the two daughters again thanked me for caring for them and for their mom. Oh yes, once again, "P.S. I made a little arrangement of flowers for you. Enjoy the chocolates too!" And I did.

Many of my patients loved bringing food into the office for me to share with office staff. There were donuts, boxes of candy, fruit baskets, and the like. It is easy to see why weight management for me has always been a challenge, all those goodies plus a love of pizza. That was a lovely thing to do; however, much nicer were the gifts of homemade delights made by my patients as they were preparing to come to see me.

One such patient that I still recall with great fondness was Kitty. That was what she was called by family and friends, although I do not think that was her given name. Kitty was a southern belle with two loving adult daughters. I first took care of Kitty around the turn of the century; I think 1997 or 1998. She had an advanced and incurable ovarian cancer. I operated on her at least twice and treated her with chemotherapy on several occasions during the six or seven years I cared for her. She was sweet and grateful, and she had a special talent for lemon bars.

I think Kitty made the best lemon bars ever. They were certainly the best lemon bars I ever tasted, even up until today. Every time she came in to see me, she brought about a dozen lemon bars wrapped in foil. As soon as I tasted one the first time, I decided that I was not going to share them with office personnel. They were too good, and I was just too selfish, not that I needed the caloric load they provided. I would eat one at home and then put them in the freezer to enjoy later. I even hid them from my kids. Whenever I wanted a real treat, I would go to the freezer and take one and only one lemon bar, defrost it and enjoy it. There were times I had Kitty come in a bit earlier than necessary to see me in the office if I was running low on those lemon bars.

Kitty and her daughters knew how much I loved them. They enjoyed bringing them to me. And then as Kitty's story was approaching its end, the family called me because she was too weak to come in to see me. They assured me that Kitty had made me some lemon bars they would bring in for me when they had a free moment. Well, Kitty died a few days after that phone call. A couple of weeks later, there were Kitty's lemon bars brought in by her daughters, made with love during her final days. I brought those treats home and at first, I just could not bring myself to eat them. But I broke down; they were too good to leave in the freezer, even though Kitty was gone. I ate one and then a week or so later, I enjoyed another. When I got to the last one, I left it in the freezer for several weeks, because I was not ready to let her go. And finally, I ate that last lemon bar, and I said my final goodbye to Kitty.

CHAPTER TWENTY-SEVEN

CONTROL AND UNCERTAINTY

Two of the most frightening things about a cancer diagnosis are the sense that one is no longer in control of their body and the uncertainty of what the future holds. Uncertainty of the future is an unsettling aspect of life. Who knows what tomorrow, next week, next month or next year has to offer? Will I be infected with COVID and if so, how will it affect my body and my life? Is my job secure, and if not, what new challenges will I face? I have a family history of dementia, what is my risk of inheriting this disease and the resulting loss of everything that defines me?

The list is endless but typically we don't dwell on life's uncertainties. We understand that uncertainty is a part of life, and that knowledge becomes a part of the white noise that always surrounds us. But when one hears that they have cancer, it is difficult to ignore the uncertainty of the future. Will I be cured? If I die, how will my family deal with my passing? Who will raise my children? One important defense mechanism to help deal with uncertainty is to be informed and to be proactive in one's own management.

This section is about autonomy. It is the ability to make decisions without the direction from others. Loss of autonomy is akin to being in prison where all decisions are taken from you and made by others.

Exercising autonomy amounts to seizing control of one's life. Being diagnosed with cancer can be likened to imprisonment with loss of control of all aspects of one's life. It doesn't have to be that way. Remember, patients, unlike prisoners, have veto power over decisions about their care. When one understands that they are the most important member of the treatment team, it should be enlightening. There is no reason for patients to blindly abdicate control of treatment decisions to one's health care providers. One should refuse to be treated until sufficiently informed about their disease and treatment options to understand the how and the why of whatever treatment is decided upon.

I have found during my career that many patients willingly give up the control they are entitled to exercise. I always tried to engage my patients in the treatment decisions by providing important information about their disease and its treatment choices. I always tried to provide information in a language that was easy to understand. I avoided using medical terms when familiar wording was possible. For example, instead of metastasis I would say cancer spread, instead of stage of disease I indicated where the cancer was located. I encouraged patients to record what I said , so they could replay our discussion if they wish. When asked, or when I felt that a patient needed to know, I offered to provide critical information about their short-term and long-term prognosis. That information should help her make critical decisions that would impact her life.

Permit me to expand that thought. Often there is more than one good treatment choice when providing cancer care. Sometimes choices include standard therapies versus clinical trials. Sometimes there is uncertainty whether one standard treatment choice is better than another. Sometimes no treatment at all is an option, especially with advanced cancer, and especially after all effective therapies have been exhausted. Sometimes therapies with possible benefits exist, but patients might be too frail to withstand such treatments. Sometimes costs enter into the equation. Sometimes a decision needs to be made about the timing of treatment. If one's cancer has recurred and is no longer curable but possibly responsive to further treatment, should one begin treatment sooner rather than later? For example, what if such a patient has long wished to travel to the city from which their family emigrated to America? And suppose that such a trip including the necessary planning would result in a delay of a month before a treatment would be started. And suppose such a delay might result in a progression of the cancer. Should the patient travel or be treated? Remember that cure is no longer on the table. Only the patient can decide; however, all too often that decision is relegated to the treatment team.

So let me share a couple of stories that illustrate the issues of this section of *Storms Passing*. I recall Zoe, a professional thirty-something woman with a husband and two small children. She presented with a large but early-stage cervical cancer. It was confined to the cervix but had expanded this normally three-centimeter organ to about six centimeters. That is a big cervical cancer! When I first met Zoe there were two equally effective treatment choices. One consisted of a radical hysterectomy with removal of the uterus, cervix and upper vagina along with the lymph nodes in the pelvis. The ovaries could be spared because cervical cancers typically do not spread to the ovaries. A woman in her thirties benefits greatly from the hormones produced by the ovaries, so their preservation is strong reason to select this approach. The surgical approach commonly results in poor bladder control which often lasts for weeks or months and can be permanent. Furthermore, with a large cancer, there was also the possible need for radiation after the surgery which would void the benefits of saving the ovaries as the radiation would destroy their function to produce hormones including estrogens. Now, if radiation was required after surgery, the risks and complications of this combined approach of surgery followed by radiation therapy would exceed that of either treatment alone.

The other treatment option was to administer weekly chemotherapy for six weeks along with radiation therapy as I described in a prior section. Surgery would not be a part of the treatment plan. This treatment approach offered an equal chance of cure to surgery but would destroy ovarian function. Furthermore, radiation therapy can result in injury to the bowel and bladder that can necessitate further surgery. Not an easy decision! So, Zoe said, as so many before her and after her, "You are the doctor, you tell me what I should do." By her instructions, she gave up her veto power and choice. I had to choose for her even though she had enough information to make the difficult decision herself. My motto is "your body, your choice" but Zoe was uncomfortable being responsible for making the decision.

As a follow-up, I did a radical hysterectomy, and she did require further radiation therapy because I found spread of the cancer to a lymph node in the pelvis, but she is cured of her disease. Fortunately, she has not had serious complications of her operation or her radiation therapy. Zoe remains on hormone replacement therapy as the radiation therapy made her menopausal. Had she opted for the radiation therapy option with chemotherapy, she would have likely had the same outcome without the need for surgery. This is not to suggest that one was a better choice than the other, only that she could have chosen either option but she gave up that control

The second patient, Bianca , is from a traditional Italian family that emigrated to the United States about thirty years ago. Bianca's immediate family included two daughters and a husband. She was sent to me with a newly diagnosed cancer of the ovary and over three years I performed surgery followed by chemotherapy. I then followed her closely for a possible recurrence of her cancer. When her cancer recurred, I wanted to tell her and discuss various options and choices that she had; however, she spoke only Italian and her family refused to allow me to tell her she had recurrent cancer. Frankly, many foreign-speaking patients accompanied by family members have similar experiences to Bianca's. Family members have explained to me that they believe that their mom or sister or whomever will give up the will to live if informed of any bad news such as a cancer recurrence. At the same time, I have found that most of these patients do understand that introduction of some new treatment after a long period without treatment means that the cancer has recurred, and they accept this information. And, they don't give up their will to live!

The result of keeping the patient in the dark in circumstances such as Bianca's is that the patient and the family never have the chance to openly discuss her treatment options, her prognosis, and the patient's wishes as her end approaches. Such a sad set of circumstances when the intention of family members is good but misdirected and the patient loses the opportunity to participate in the decision-making for her cancer treatment.

The third patient, Martha, went about this whole process differently than Zoe and Bianca. . She also had an advanced ovarian cancer that recurred. She had a family history of both breast and ovarian cancer and genetic testing showed that she was BRCA 1 positive. I had operated on her, had given her chemotherapy following surgery. I had treated her again after her cancer recurred two years later. She had a second recurrence after being free of cancer for another year. So, we discussed her options which included trying different chemotherapy drugs or starting on a clinical trial of what was a new drug at the time, Olaparib. Olaparib is a PARP inhibitor which is a type of targeted therapy. Early trials had shown that BRCA positive patients with ovarian cancers often had good responses to this drug. Martha had several questions about the choices. She wanted to know about toxicity and response rates for both options. She wanted to know how many patients had been treated with Olaparib and whether any had died of complications. She was interested in any information she could read about Olaparib, and I gave her information about the clinical trials to review. She actually contacted the principal investigator for the most recent of the trials to find out what other patients had experienced. She went home, did some outside reading and returned, excited to try the new drug. She actually had a remarkable response after initiating the Olaparib and remained free of disease when I retired. While not likely cured, she has clearly benefited from this process and felt in control of her choices.

I hope I never get cancer, but if I do, I know I will be in control like Martha, not Zoe or Bianca. Maintaining control is empowering and should always be pursued by the patient. Sometimes a doctor does not provide enough information for a patient to feel as if she is a participant in the decision-making process. Sometimes a doctor is unwilling to provide the time needed to answer questions of a patient and her family. When a doctor doesn't feel comfortable with discussing these issues with the patient or doesn't have the time, I believe that is not the right doctor to provide for her care.

CHAPTER TWENTY-EIGHT

FINAL WORDS : THE DIFFICULT END-OF-LIFE DISCUSSION

In writing this book I was often reminded of the many times in my career I sat with my patients who were nearing the end-of-life. These moments are never easy for the physician and even worse for the patient and her family, but they are very important. What techniques did I employ in counseling my patients who are dying?

First, I believed that my patients and their family members deserved to be told what I knew about their prognosis as the end approached. It is never advisable to be precise about the future because the short-term future is always uncertain, and some patients live weeks or months longer or fewer than one might anticipate. I might say, instead, "while it is never possible to state with confidence how much time you might have, based on my experience I believe that we are in the final weeks or final months." (A patient with a bowel blockage would typically be in her final weeks or even days while a long-standing patient with slowly progressive cancer after exhausting all available options would typically be in her final months). In my experience, I found that patients approaching end-of-life were already acutely aware of the unfavorable prognosis and understood that the end was near. I also found that they usually have accepted this and are at peace, knowing that they gave their all in a battle that is now over.

Second, I encouraged my patient to have family members with her at these times because even though *they* might have been at peace and accepting their poor prognosis and limited life expectancy, family members often were not so accepting. Furthermore, families often wanted their loved one to continue the fight even after any realistic hope of prolongation of life had passed. Knowledgeable physicians know that this thinking can only be harmful to the patient who is trying to move on and prepare herself for her passing.

I have seen patients agree to follow the wishes of their family members, often resulting in painful and expensive ventures. Sometimes these fruitless efforts have taken patients to Mexico, the Philippines, or other venues where unscrupulous individuals offered hope when no likelihood of significant prolongation or improved quality of life remained. "Therapies" in these circumstances are typically offered so long as the patient or her family can pay or until they finally see the futility of continuing this harmful pathway.

I can illustrate how devastating this pathway can be by sharing a story of one of my patients who was also a friend. She died from advanced ovarian cancer several years ago. Prior to her death, at a time that her quality of life was good although her prognosis for long term survival was poor, her husband developed an aggressive cancer in the lungs that progressed rapidly. How much tragedy can one family endure? As his condition progressed over several months to the point that breathing was becoming difficult for him, he went to Mexico for unproven and untested therapies. These efforts bought him neither more time nor improved his quality of life. These "therapies" depleted much of their savings as is typical of such treatments.

Furthermore, both he and his wife lost the opportunity to deal effectively with issues that are so important as one approaches the end-of-life. And when he passed, *my* patient with cancer had to deal with the financial burden of his "alternative treatments." She did this alone while grieving and having to fight her own battle with cancer.

Frankly, I have seen many physicians continue to offer cancer therapies after it is clear that further treatment with more chemotherapy, surgery or radiation therapy will no longer offer palliation of symptoms or prolongation of life. This is done in an effort to "never give up." But in reality, in my opinion, it is a defense mechanism of the doctor to avoid discussing end-of-life issues with the patient. When, for example, the chance of a short-term benefit is a 5% possibility of prolonging a poor quality of life by a month or two and the risk of significant side effects of treatment is close to 100%, it is time to stop therapy and begin counselling the patient as I am detailing.

Let me use ovarian cancer to emphasize this point. We know that most patients present with advanced cancers. We also know that the best initial treatment is a combination of surgery and drug therapy. The drugs typically are chemotherapy drugs often in conjunction with newer biological therapies (e.g., PARP inhibitors, antiangiogenic drugs, etc.) We also know that a small percentage of such patients are actually cured of their cancers, but most will experience a recurrence of their cancers. When those cancers recur, they often will respond to further drug therapies, but inevitably, almost all of those who respond will have further recurrences. At this point often a third treatment is offered, and some patients will respond for a time to this; however, the percentage of responders is much less and the duration of the responses is typically much shorter. At some point in time, perhaps after a fourth or even a fifth treatment intervention, it should be obvious that further therapy buys toxicity without realistic chance of benefit. Furthermore, at that time, patients are usually symptomatic and frankly exhausted from her therapies. That is when end-of-life discussion should be undertaken. Instead, I have seen patients receiving 6th or 7th or 8th or more different types of treatments without any measurable benefit in such cases!

When I plan to discuss end-of-life issues with a patient, either between just the two of us or, preferably, with her family, first I ask permission to initiate the discussion. I might say "I know that you have been having a really difficult time these past months with your treatments and I haven't been able to give you much good news along the way. I wonder if this is a good time for us to discuss my thoughts?"

I am prepared for her to say "Not right now, doctor," in which case I will suggest that we might set aside some time in the near future. More commonly, my patient will understand that this is an important chance to discuss much of what she has been thinking lately and importantly a chance to get the family on board with her prognosis.

If my patient gives me permission to hold this meeting with her and her family, I make certain that there will be no interruptions from the operating room or from my clinic. I turn off my telephone and I sit down near my patient. It is important to sit, not stand. Standing would be more intimidating to everyone in attendance and often would suggest that I am in a hurry. I am not giving a lecture. I am sharing information with my patient. We meet in a conference room or private office, if possible, not at a hospital bedside. We sit as friends do when sharing information. It's a two-way street.

For most patients I start the discussion by briefly recalling her experiences as my patient. "I remember when I first met you at my office after your doctor sent you to me with that large mass in your abdomen. I suspected ovarian cancer and ran several tests that confirmed my suspicion. So, we discussed a plan of management that likely would include surgery and chemotherapy, and in fact, that is exactly what we did. Our hopes were really high, but we knew that these cancers are very dangerous because they often are advanced when they are diagnosed. You recall that your cancer was stage III-C which is typical for cancers of the ovaries. As we discussed at the time, the outcome is uncertain at the time of diagnosis. Now here we are, and you did really well for two years before your cancer came back. You lost your hair, but it grew back. During that time, you were able to enjoy your family and do the things you enjoy doing. We tried other treatments that helped some but not as much as we had hoped. I know that these past few months have been really hard on you. You have lost a lot of weight and are having a hard time finding the energy to do the things you really enjoy doing. I can see that, and you have shared as much with me."

All of this preamble to the subject material of end-of-life is to educate my patient's family and to give her a little time to compose herself. She invariably understands where the conversation is going, and both welcomes and dreads it. But the discussion is important. She knows that. This is a good opportunity for my patient to ask questions. Often family members will chime in with thoughts or questions of their own. It is so important that everyone in the room knows that this meeting is important for my patient and that there is no rush to finish the meeting. Since I take care of patients in the academic setting with residents and fellows, sometimes one and only one trainee will be in the room during the discussion, but that individual is only an observer and does not enter into any dialogue.

The content of the dialogue itself must be honest, respectful, and direct. There should be no confusion about the meaning of what I am saying. I might acknowledge that there are other therapies but, unfortunately, they offer little hope of prolonging her life.

And they will surely adversely impact the quality of her life. I might acknowledge that some patients elect to try other treatments, but I discourage them because when considering the risk versus the benefit, minimal if any benefit is outweighed by the certainty of adverse side effects in this situation.

I always support a request for another opinion, and when requested I will direct my patient to high-quality physicians, typically in an academic medical setting. In Southern California those recommendations would include UCLA, University of Southern California, Cedars Sinai Medical Center, and the City of Hope. These are all NCI (National Cancer Institute) designated Cancer Centers, recognized for their excellence in cancer care throughout the world. I acknowledge that there are other practitioners in the area who also have a lot of experience in caring for patients with advanced cancers; however, I emphasize that I recommend individuals in centers that are widely recognized for their expertise in caring for such patients. I also reassure my patient that I will be happy to continue caring for her if she decides to obtain other opinions and then wishes to return to my care.

I attempt to offer my thoughts and opinions in as kind and as sensitive a manner as possible. I invite questions or thoughts throughout the discussion period. The hope that I offer is for my patient to be as comfortable as possible and to be able to engage with family and friends during her remaining time. I always emphasize that, just as I have been her treating physician when surgery or chemotherapy was indicated, I will continue to be actively involved in her care without active treatment. I will not abandon her and will always be there for her.

This commitment then typically leads to a discussion of management of symptoms associated with advanced cancers which might include pain, nausea, vomiting, fatigue, anxiety, and depression. I will discuss the role of pain management teams who are uniquely trained in managing pain if they have not already been a part of her treatment team. The goal of pain management is to provide comfort without excessive sedation; a tricky balancing act that pain management physicians are remarkably effective in accomplishing. I discuss the role of home health and hospice care in an effort to help her keep comfortable and out of the hospital. At these times, most patients prefer to be in the home rather than in a hospital. This information can be invaluable to my patients. I offer the support of social services to help coordinate management of their symptoms and home healthcare. There are psychologists and social workers who are particularly effective at counseling patients at the end of their lives. I provide that information to them at this time, if requested.

And I hug my patient. I always hug my patient. I want her to know she is special to me and that our relationship is more than just patient and doctor. She is a friend. I continue to want the best for her. When the session comes to a close, I do not say goodbye or it has been my honor to care for you, rather I say, "I will see you soon." Or "Our journey together is not at an end." Those words confirm my commitment to helping provide for her care rather than a promise that I will actually see her again. And I invite her to contact me if there are questions or concerns she has moving forward. I shake hands with her family if I have not met them previously. I hug them if I know them from their participation in her care over the months and years. And we say goodbye, for now.

VERY BRIEF EPILOGUE

This marks the end of my narrative. I didn't expect to write so much, but I loved reliving some of the experiences I have shared in this book. Since I have kept the notes sent to me from patients over the years of my practice, it was an easy task to include them verbatim in the stories I have told. I have shared the content of the book with some of the patients whose stories I have told. I am grateful to them for what has been uniformly positive feedback. The book provides a mix of stories along with some personal philosophy and a lot of my background that I didn't include in my autobiography which I wrote for my family and which I have not chosen to publish.

The women whose stories I have told had gynecologic cancers. All of them feared the possibility of dying from their disease. It is easy to view their cancer as evil; however, cancer is merely a part of life. Cancer is experienced by some but touches almost everyone at some point in their lives through their own illness or that of family members or friends. Elie Wiesel, a Holocaust survivor and Nobel laureate, once said that "Indifference to me, is the epitome of all evil." It is worse than hate. But he was not speaking of cancer or other natural diseases as being evil. Rather he was speaking of evil deeds by men or society to others. A more apt statement relevant to the care of oncology patients is "Indifference to suffering is evil." I hold that belief in my heart. I hope I have never been indifferent to the suffering of my patients.

I also hope that sharing personal notes and cards sent to me by my patients is not viewed as being boastful or lacking in humility. That was not my purpose even though the content of many of these notes seem self-serving and self-aggrandizing. I wanted to give the reader a sense of the difference one can make in the lives of others through personal commitment and hard work. I also wanted to demonstrate that expressions of gratitude toward others is truly a gift that enriches the giver and the recipient. I have certainly been enriched by the expressions of gratitude and love from so many of my patients.

All my patients were women whom I didn't know until they were sent to me for care. All of them were frightened yet hopeful of a favorable outcome. They relied on me to provide them with confidence that they were in good hands and that I would be there for them, whatever their medical needs might be. I tried to accomplish this by being sensitive to their fears, knowledgeable about their disease, and respectful of their privacy and their self-worth.

At times I also needed to be there for their psychosocial needs, and, to the best of my abilities, I tried to fill that role as well. I tried to care for them honestly, benevolently, and always respectful of their humanity. I was not perfect, but I like to believe that I was very good as a physician and as a role model for others.

In return for my efforts, my patients provided me with a life full of purpose, responsibility and a sense of self-worth. I believe in behaving honestly, performing kind acts, being compassionate, grateful, loving and forgiving. I have tried to meet those goals professionally and personally. Finally, I have tried to set an example for those I trained through my deeds and my words. I hope those who have known me would say I have met those worthy goals.

Michael L. Berman, MD, FACOG

NOTES TO MY READERS:

About the foreward: by Dr Tewari: *A Meaningful Life,* was composed over the course of four days during early March 2021 on the outside patio at the Bahia Corinthian Yacht Club in Newport Beach, California.

About the cover: In these pages there is a patient named Zahra whose story is shared. Several years after her recurrent cancer had been treated successfully, she expressed interest in obtaining an image Dr. Berman created entitled *Storm Brewing* photographed in 2015 in Antarctica, one year after his wife's passing. He suggested that, in Zahra's case, the title could be changed to *Storm Passed* given her favorable outcome. He thought this image should grace the cover of the book to symbolize the many storms weathered by his patients, some of which still rage.

It is this spirit in which the book title, *Storms Passing,* has been chosen.

Acknowledgments

There are many individuals to whom I owe a debt of gratitude in encouraging me to write this book and in helping to bring this project, first envisioned during Covid in 2020, to publication. My girlfriend, Bonnie Marcus, was getting tired of my looking for things to keep me occupied since our travel was severely curtailed by this epidemic. She encouraged me to "write something" and get out from under foot. That led to my drafting my autobiography and then, the following year, a draft I entitled Storms Passing. While writing this book, Bonnie served as my sounding board. As a retired social worker, she helped me direct much of the dialogue to the psychosocial aspects of patient care, which is the theme of this writing.

I also want to thank my former resident who became my gynecologic oncology fellow and then my colleague at the University of California, Irvine, Dr Krishnansu Tewari, for his encouragement and for writing the foreward to Storms Passing. Krish is a remarkably creative and gifted individual with interests in the arts as well as the sciences. He has tireless energy as he continues to train residents and fellows, cares for his patients, writes manuscripts for scientific publications, and directs much of the research in gynecologic oncology at the University of California, Irvine. Thankfully, some of that energy was directed towards this effort, and I am grateful to him.

I am most grateful to my friend, Rick Taylor, whom I met while on a ship traveling the Beagle Channel between Argentina and Chile earlier this year. Rick shared with me that he had written a book entitled *This Eternity* which was published recently. I told him that I had also written a manuscript for my friends and family to read. When I mentioned the content and theme of the manuscript, he expressed interest in seeing it. I sent him the e-file which he read and enjoyed. He mentioned a very positive experience with his publisher, Rip Coleman of Bohannon Hall Press in publishing his book and asked if I would allow him to share my manuscript with Rip. I was excited when both Rick and Rip were enthusiastic about the content and supported my publishing it with Bohannon Hall Press.

With Rip's guidance and suggestions, I rewrote and expanded the original document to its current content. Without Rick's encouragement and editing skills and Rip's support and publishing skills, this effort would not have resulted in its publication. I am so grateful to both of them for their encouragement and support throughout the writing and publishing process.

I would be remiss if I didn't thank my children, who from time to time over the years, asked "How was your day, dad." This book was written to answer that question and also to provide guidance to their children, my grand-children, as they move forward with their lives.

Finally, and most importantly, I thank my patients for the honor of trusting me with their lives when they were most vulnerable and threatened. And I am so grateful to them for teaching me how I should live my life. They taught me about hope and love and compassion and strength in the face of profound adversity. Their stories and lessons provide the foundation for this book and, more importantly to me, showed me how to become the person I wanted to be.

Sources cited in the Foreward:

1. *The Tyger* by William Blake (1794).
2. Zohar: Primary text of Kabbalah—Moses de León (1240-1305).
3. Rolling Stones Steel Wheels/Urban Jungle Tour (1989)
4. *Memories and Stories: 1942-2020* by Michael L Berman, MD (2020).
5. *Moksha Patamu* (Snakes & Ladders)—game based on morality invented by Hindu spiritual teachers (16th Century).
6. *Three Turnings of the Wheel of Dharma, Indus Valley Civilization* (2500 BCE)
7. *Blood on the Tracks*—15th studio album by Bob Dylan (1975)
8. *Wondrous Stories* by Jon Anderson,
   song from the studio album *Going for the One by Yes* (1977).
9. *Thus Spoke Zarathustra: A Book for All and None*
   by Friedrich Nietzsche (1883-1885)
10. *The Psychopathology of Everyday Life* by Sigmund Freud (1904)
11. *Memories, dreams, Reflections* by Carl Jung (1962)
12. *Saving Private Ryan*, directed by Steven Spielberg (1998)
13. *Songs of Innocence and of Experience* by William Blake (1789)
14. *Jerusalem* by William Blake (1804)
15. *Storm Brewing,* photograph by Dr. Michael L Berman (2015)

Made in the USA
Monee, IL
12 November 2026

813f147d-2c81-4b4d-a2c9-32b900208bb9R01